Applied Yoga™ for Musculoskeletal Pain

of related interest

Pain Science – Yoga – Life
Bridging Neuroscience and Yoga for Pain Care
Marnie Hartman and Niamh Moloney
Forewords by Tiffany Cruikshank and Gwendolen Jull
ISBN 978 1 91208 558 3
eISBN 978 1 91208 562 0

Yoga and Science in Pain Care
Treating the Person in Pain
Edited by Neil Pearson, Shelly Prosko and Marlysa Sullivan
Foreword by Timothy McCall
ISBN 978 1 84819 397 0
eISBN 978 0 85701 354 5

Trauma-Informed Yoga for Pain Management
A Practical Manual for Simple Stretching, Gentle Strengthening, and Mindful Breathing
Yael Calhoun with Mona Bingham
ISBN 978 1 83997 800 5
eISBN 978 1 83997 801 2

Yoga for Sports Performance
A Guide for Yoga Therapists, Yoga Teachers and Bodyworkers
Jim Harrington
ISBN 978 1 84819 406 9
eISBN 978 0 85701 362 0

APPLIED YOGA™ FOR MUSCULOSKELETAL PAIN

Integrating Yoga, Physical Therapy, Strength, and Spirituality

JORY SEROTA, C-IAYT, LMT, NKT

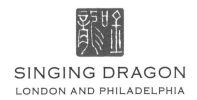

SINGING DRAGON
LONDON AND PHILADELPHIA

First published in Great Britain in 2024 by Singing Dragon,
an imprint of Jessica Kingsley Publishers
Part of John Murray Press

1

Copyright © Jory Serota 2024

The right of Jory Serota to be identified as the Author of the Work has been asserted
by him in accordance with the Copyright, Designs and Patents Act 1988.

Photography copyright © Aigul Moon Photography and Kritchathorn Charumar 2024
Illustrations copyright © Simon Ampel 2024

Front cover image source: Aigul Moon Photography. The cover image is
for illustrative purposes only, and any person featuring is a model.

All rights reserved. No part of this publication may be reproduced, stored in
a retrieval system, or transmitted, in any form or by any means without the
prior written permission of the publisher, nor be otherwise circulated in any
form of binding or cover other than that in which it is published and without
a similar condition being imposed on the subsequent purchaser.

A CIP catalogue record for this title is available from the
British Library and the Library of Congress

ISBN 978 1 83997 882 1
eISBN 978 1 83997 883 8

Printed and bound in the United States by Integrated Books International

Jessica Kingsley Publishers' policy is to use papers that are natural, renewable and recyclable
products and made from wood grown in sustainable forests. The logging and manufacturing
processes are expected to conform to the environmental regulations of the country of origin.

Singing Dragon
Carmelite House
50 Victoria Embankment
London EC4Y 0DZ

www.singingdragon.com

John Murray Press
Part of Hodder & Stoughton Limited
An Hachette UK Company

Contents

Part I: Embodiment and the Path to Freedom

Introduction: The Beginnings of Applied Yoga™ 9

1. Yoga in the West. 13
   Yoga for Chronic Pain 16
   The Rise of Injuries in Yoga 19
   Yoga and Mental Health 24
   Is Yoga Spiritual? 26
   Being in the Body 27
   The Psychosomatic Experience 29
   Techniques for Releasing Emotional Tension 31
   Spiritual Bypassing 34

2. Principles of Sports Conditioning 45
   Types of Muscles 49
   Types of Muscular Contractions 50
   Muscle Strains 51
   Tendon Injuries 52
   The RICE Myth 53
   Good Pain vs. Bad Pain 56
   Kinesiophobia: Fear of Movement 58
   What is Stretching? 59
   Types of Stretching 60
   The Stretch Reflex 62
   How Long to Stretch For 63
   Stretching for Athletes 66

3. The Breath 71
   History of Pranayama 72
   The Breath and the Nervous System 73

The Diaphragm	77
Diaphragmatic and Thoracic Breathing	78
Breathing and Athletic Performance	80
Nasal Breathing vs. Mouth Breathing	80
Guidelines for Working with the Breath	82
Where in the Body to Breathe?	83
The Breathwork Practice: Learning to Breathe into the Body	83
A Tip on Meditation from the Buddha	90
Types of Pranayamas	90
Which Pranayama to Practice?	93
When to Practice	93
A Note on One Other Form of Breathwork: Holotropic Breathwork	93
Breathwork and Asana Practice	94

Part II: Applying the Teachings: The Movement Practices

4. Anatomy of the Lower Back 101

Low Back Sequence Part I: Weeks 1 and 2   105

Low Back Sequence Part II: Weeks 3 and 4   110

5. Anatomy of the Hip. 119

Hip Sequence Part I: Weeks 1 and 2   121

Hip Sequence Part II: Weeks 3 and 4   128

6. Anatomy of the Knee. 139

Knee Sequence Part I: Weeks 1 and 2   142

Knee Sequence Part II: Weeks 3 and 4   148

7. Anatomy of the Shoulder 153

Shoulder Sequence Part I: Weeks 1 and 2   155

Shoulder Sequence Part II: Weeks 3 and 4   161

8. Anatomy of the Neck. 169

Neck Sequence   173

9. Bonus Section: Sacroiliac Joint and Glute Strength 197

Glute Sequence: Weeks 1–3   198

Endnotes 203

Index. 217

Acknowledgments 224

PART I

EMBODIMENT AND THE PATH TO FREEDOM

Introduction: The Beginnings of Applied Yoga™

I began practicing yoga at the ripe age of 18, but not for the reason you might think. There were no spiritual intentions involved in my decision to take up the practice, even though it would later become the guiding philosophy of my life.

I grew up as an athlete, specifically playing baseball and tennis. During my senior year of high school, I played second singles while my best friend played first. I was better than him, but he had seniority, playing the previous five years, so our coach gave him the head honor. He and I would compete at most things throughout high school, a trend that lasts to this day.

We spoke on the phone one night during our second semester in college—me at Florida State and he at NYU—and he told me he was going to start yoga. My first thought was "There's no way you're going to do yoga and not me." The next day, I went to a class at my local gym and completely fell in love. My body moved in ways it had never moved before, and when I left, I felt like I was walking on a cloud.

The emotions that dominated my childhood—anger, fear, insecurity—were nonexistent. I felt as if I could connect with anyone, look people in the eye, and even talk to a woman if the opportunity arose.

I thought to myself, "If one class made me feel this good, I wonder what a life of it would do?" I woke up at six the next morning and began practicing what I remembered of the sun salutation. My path was set.

My friend?

He never made it to class. He did eventually do a teacher training program and lived in a yoga studio, but he never took to it as I did. His influence on me, however, cannot be forgotten, and I will forever be grateful for it.

Yoga was introduced to me with many promises, the first of those being increased flexibility. At the time I started practicing, I was playing ultimate frisbee for Florida State and quickly found that the daily classes were increasing my athleticism on the field. Our team was ranked in the nation's top 15, and within months I rose to become the number-three player on the team.

As the years progressed and I moved away from playing ultimate frisbee, I began to see the impact my practice had on every aspect of my life, bringing forth a strength I could always sense was there but hadn't experienced yet.

On my 22nd birthday, I found myself in Rishikesh, India, widely considered to be the yoga capital of the world. I had been traveling through Southeast Asia for nearly nine months and had heard of a Romanian Swami that *I had* to study with. I rejected that idea quickly, believing I did not travel to India to study with a foreigner, but after hearing his name again and again, I decided to take a class and was immediately mesmerized by his teachings.

Swami taught me that yoga goes much deeper than the asana practice, or the physical yoga postures. He taught about chakras, concentrating the mind, withdrawing the senses, and entering the higher stages of the yogic path. His talks, normally to a room of 100 eager students, were some of the most inspiring moments I'd ever had. His teacher training program was 36 intensive months. I stayed for two months and it changed my life.

Before going to India, I had been practicing around an hour a day, but that quickly turned into two. By the time I returned to the United States, a fire had been lit under me and I began to spend a minimum of three to four hours a day on my mat—sometimes even reaching six or seven. This level of dedication lasted nearly six years. I was determined to understand the tradition, both its physical and esoteric aspects.

In 2002, I discovered Iyengar yoga and a teacher named Glenn Black who ignited my love for human biomechanics. I had been practicing long holds of each posture from what I was taught in India, but I had not received specific directions on how to maintain joint health and tissue integrity. The alignment principles and attention to detail that Iyengar yoga expounded were insightful. My practice continued to range between two and four hours every day, this time with a much greater focus on anatomy than it had before.

I found that by practicing this way, my body was getting stronger, and little aches and pains were disappearing. When something would catch in my hip or back, I would give it attention in my practice, make minor adjustments to whatever pose I was in, and offer myself a very specific and effective form of physical therapy. There was nothing that could arise in my body that I didn't have the confidence I could heal with yoga.

As my practice became an integrated part of my life over the years, my body continued to strengthen. A new vitality was awakening in me. Instead of insecurity, I developed physical, spiritual, and psychological confidence. I was becoming a different person.

I am beyond grateful for the effects yoga has had on my life. From self-empowerment and knowledge to giving me a career, it has been one of my life's strongest and most valuable relationships.

Many of the promises the yoga world made to me, however, never came true.

I found that increasing flexibility does not necessarily translate into less pain—a topic we will discuss in great depth throughout this book. Standing on my head for 20 minutes a day will not prevent male pattern baldness; on the other hand, developing physical strength, something yoga does not proficiently speak about at all, aids in protecting our muscles as well as healing them after an injury.

My mission for years now has been to synthesize the wisdom of the asana practice with the science of movement. The balance between yoga and physical therapy, flexibility and strength, spirituality and humanness has fueled me and helped to shape my understanding of the human body, the way that I teach, the therapy I perform, and the creation of Applied Yoga™.

CHAPTER 1

Yoga in the West

Yoga is traditionally a physical, mental, and spiritual practice which originated in India more than 2500 years ago. The word "yoga" comes from the Sanskrit word *yuj*, meaning "to join," and symbolizes the union of the body, mind, and spirit.

In Patanjali's *Yoga Sutra*, one of the first and most important texts on yoga, he states that there are eight limbs to the yogic path. Each limb represents a specific stage that is to be progressed through until one attains enlightenment.

These eight limbs are:

1. yama (social and ethical guidelines)
2. niyama (personal spiritual practices)
3. asana (physical postures)
4. pranayama (breath control and energy management)
5. pratyahara (sense withdrawal)
6. dharana (concentration)
7. dhyana (meditation)
8. samadhi (enlightenment).

In the West, yoga has come to mainly be a combination of asana and pranayama techniques aimed at making the body feel better and increasing happiness. It is taught in yoga studios, gyms, spas, corporate offices, community centers, personal homes, and online. The spiritual aspects of the practice are regularly mocked, with commercials that have yogis eating a slice of pizza while in a pose or TV shows where the teacher is egregiously over-spiritual and not really connected to a sense of reality. This is not far off the mark for how some classes are presented and it can be quite a turn-off for those hoping to find respite from life's daily grind. Teachers will tell their students to "melt their hearts" (whatever that means) and present a spacy, airy demeanor as opposed to something rooted in mindfulness and attention.

13

The number-one reason people begin practicing yoga today is increased flexibility.[1] Yoga can provide a physical freedom not offered by many other modalities, and people are able to very quickly have a different experience of their bodies than they have been used to. What's interesting about this, though, is that the majority of people who do begin for physical reasons continue going to class because of the effect on their personal development and ability to manage stress.[2] This shows that the underlying, inherent spirituality of yoga practice supports mental health and is the primary reason so many practitioners remain devoted to it for many years.

Although yoga has been known in India for millennia, it wasn't until the 1980s and 1990s that it began to make a significant impact on the West. It was different from the weight training we had known with superstars such as Lou Ferrigno and Arnold Schwarzenegger. Yoga was a path to enlightenment, inner peace, and true physical freedom. Yoga teachers espoused that by bending and pushing your body in these unique ways, you could alleviate discomfort, awaken youthfulness, and increase longevity.

A lot of that was true, and the glowing testimonials were pouring in. Yoga was healing chronic back aches and fixing knee problems. Students were finding a new range of motion in their joints and flexibility in their muscles. Many of them felt physically and emotionally freer than they ever had before.

In many ways, however, these Western yogis were test dummies for intensive group practice. Yoga was traditionally learned in a one-on-one setting between guru (teacher) and shishya (student). Sri Krishnamacarya, to whom we owe most of our knowledge of yoga, was taught in this manner and passed the lineage down to his son T.K.V. Desikachar, and also B.K.S. Iyengar and Pattabhi Jois among others. It's quite possible, actually, that Iyengar taught the first ever public yoga class in 1937 when Krishnamacarya sent him to Pune, India, to spread yoga. Iyengar also brought his personal interpretation of the practice to England in 1954 through his relationship with the famous violinist Yehudi Menuhin.

In the United States, although Paramahansa Yogananda gave a powerful speech at the World Religions Council in 1893 and Sri Yogendra opened an outpost for his Indian Yoga Institute in 1920,[3] it wasn't until another student of Krishnamacarya, Indra Devi, opened her Los Angeles studio in 1948 that yoga asana became more well known. She taught a very gentle and relaxing practice that was aimed mostly at stress relief, much different from most of the yoga we know today.

MYTH BUST #1

THE MORE FLEXIBLE YOU GET, THE LESS PAIN YOU'LL HAVE AND THE CLOSER YOU'LL BE TO ENLIGHTENMENT

As the market for yoga grew, so did the commercialization. In the 1980s, Iyengar, Ashtanga, and Baptiste Power Yoga were at the forefront, and by the mid- to late 1990s, new vinyasa lineages along with Bikram and Jivamukti yoga emerged. All these styles focused very intensely on the physical practice.

The Western body is built differently to that of the Indian sage, and natural levels of flexibility between cultures varies greatly. New yogis were commonly being asked to push and stretch their bodies to areas they'd never been. Unaware of their own physical limitations, many began to overstretch their ligaments, force their joints into unnatural positions, and hurt themselves in ways they didn't realize in the moment.

Pattabhi Jois, the founder of Ashtanga yoga (who later would be accused of sexual misconduct in his classes[4]), used to say, "Practice and all is coming." Students were encouraged to push through any resistance or pain they had in a pose because yoga was a healing modality, and their pain would soon transform into freedom. It was by pushing their body to these great lengths that emancipation from suffering was claimed to arise. Many of them suffered significant injuries from this physically uneducated approach.

It has been claimed that Bikram Choudhury, an accused rapist,[5] would often forcefully push his students into poses or call them an array of derogatory names to manipulate them into going deeper into a pose. Although some of his students said that was exactly what they needed at the time, many also got hurt—both physically and emotionally—by going further than their body allowed.

Glenn Black, my first mentor of both yoga and body work, stopped teaching asana after 30 years because of the number of injuries he consistently saw from repetitive stress, overuse, and yoga-induced hypermobility. Old yogi friends of his were getting hip replacements, and he eventually had his own set of serious yoga-created injuries to deal with.

I also quickly fell prey to the "flexibility is king" thinking. I pushed myself as hard as I could, continually trusting that the more flexible I got, the better I'd feel about myself and the healthier I'd be. I practiced four hours a day for years, sometimes even seven or eight. The more I practiced, the more I tricked myself into believing I was more flexible than I was. I was never inflexible, but I certainly don't have the body of a dancer or gymnast. I soon found it would be easy to push myself too far.

In November 2015, I was living in Costa Rica and working my way into two of the deepest back bends in the yoga system. One fateful morning, I woke up with a 104°F (40°C) fever and back pain like I'd never had before. I had contracted dengue fever, which was spreading through our village. I spent the next ten days in bed watching movies and drinking water.

Dengue's nickname is the bone-crushing disease, and when it finally passed through my system and my energy returned, the back pain remained. None of my usual asana practices were effective at relieving it. It took months of therapy to feel safe again. The back pain now is nothing like it was, thanks to the low back sequence in this book, but to this day I am still not sure if the pain was caused specifically by the dengue or if I was predisposed to it from excessive back bending.

This was a pivotal moment in my life. I was more flexible than I'd ever been and, at the same time, was in more pain. The promise that flexibility equated to physical ease had failed. My body hurt. My mind was confused. My life was in a shambles. It felt like I was going through a divorce.

I lost all desire to complete the advanced yoga poses and eventually stopped practicing many of the classical ones as well. I developed a keen interest in understanding joint mechanics and human movement—concepts I already thought I had mastered but clearly hadn't.

Glenn had warned me of this, and I had seen my other most influential teacher get bilateral hip replacements in his 60s after struggling for nearly two decades. My attachment to the psychospiritual benefits I received from the practice prevented me from believing this would happen to me, especially in my late 30s. It's only now that research is proving that adverse effects often occur in yoga teachers and advanced yogis who practice more intensely and more often than others.[6]

I was determined not to leave the practice, however, but to adjust it and use it as therapy. The key to this lay not in flexibility but in the development of strength.

Yoga for Chronic Pain

Chronic pain is the leading cause of disability in the developed world and eventually progresses to decreased quality of life, depression, lack of exercise, and loss of paid work. Dissociation between body and mind occurs when people are in pain and don't have an adequate skill set for how to handle and process it. Doctors frequently overprescribe opioids which numb the pain but don't address the root cause.[7]

Yoga has a unique capacity to work with chronic pain. It can bring life force to a body that is stiff, joy to someone who is depressed, and ease to someone's physical discomfort. It is now being classified as a complementary and alternative medicine (CAM). A CAM is defined as a "group of diverse medical and health care sytems, practices, and products that are not presently considered part of conventional medicine."[8] Other examples of CAMS are massage therapy, Pilates, and acupuncture. It was estimated in 2016 that around 33.2 percent of adults have used one form of CAM in the last 12 months.[9] I suspect that number has grown significantly since then.

Yoga is adaptable and, for many people, enjoyable. It incorporates core strengthening, flexibility training, stabilization, balance, and mental health techniques. Consequently, it is finally being recommended by more doctors and frequently used by physical therapists. A single pose can address joint alignment and muscular function throughout the entire body. *Virabhadrasana II* (warrior II), for example, is commonly thought of as a pose to strengthen the quadriceps and glutes. But when practiced with astute alignment, it can work on the back foot arch, the back leg's ankle and knee, the position of the femoral head, control of the torso over the legs, the interplay between the neck and the thoracic spine, as well as the front leg's hip, knee, and ankle. Instead of simply providing therapy to an individual area as classically done, the relationship of the injured joint to the surrounding tissues can be explored.

Research in therapeutic yogic intervention is growing, as is the evidence of its effectiveness on chronic pain. Specifically designed Iyengar yoga programs decrease back pain, disability, and depression.[10] Viniyoga, a therapeutic practice created by Gary Kraftsow, has been proven more effective than cardiovascular/aerobic exercise and the use of *The Back Pain Helpbook* in decreasing pain and lack of mobility.[11] When compared to traditional exercise, hatha yoga has been shown to be more effective at improving walking pain, flexion, swelling, crepitus, and disability in patients with knee osteoarthritis,[12] as well as increasing grip strength and decreasing pain in patients with carpal tunnel syndrome.[13] Tailored yoga programs based on the Kripalu tradition show significant improvements in fatigue, energy levels, mood, and pain catastrophizing in female patients with fibromyalgia.[14]

The physical practice of yoga has another benefit: decreased opioid use. In a randomized trial for military veterans with chronic low back pain, opioid use decreased significantly.[15] This was the result of a reduction in pain and an increase in functional musculoskeletal ability.

Although there is no definitive evidence, most opioid use is the result of physical pain combined with a lack of understanding of what to do about it.

Many people freeze when pain arises and try not to move for fear of making it worse. This rarely works, and when their pain does get worse, or at least doesn't get better, the quick-fix approach is to pop a pill, get a shot, or look for a way to numb the problem.

We need to help educate people, teach them to take responsibility for what they are feeling, and guide them towards implementing an effective holistic approach. This strategy takes more time and energy, but it addresses the issue head on and gives the individual autonomy over their own body.

Many opioid users also have their identity wrapped around "being a person who's in pain," and should their pain decrease and medication change, fear exists about what they would do—especially if their pain ever comes back. This is a very complex situation involving human psychology and one's attitude towards life's difficulties. Patient education, a safe container, and various other forms of support are needed if we are to help someone in pain undertake an entirely new approach to life.

Physical pain can also cause someone to disconnect from their body. Many people "live in their heads" while working too hard and ignoring what is going on inside them. One of the many benefits that yogis report after practicing is a sense of coming home to the body. It's as though they've remembered where they are in space and now have the capacity to feel both the positive and negative sensations within their cells. This psycho-physical reconnection has been linked with improved awareness of sensory feedback and more effective motor commands to the muscles. This increase in motor ability then creates a reduction in pain, muscle tension, and spasm.[16]

Yoga also has the capacity to produce behavioral changes. A core concept within the Mahasi Sayadaw Vipassana meditation lineage states that it is not our experience that causes our suffering but our attitude towards it. This has been supported by psychotherapists and other mental health practitioners worldwide. The same can true be for physical pain. Yoga often gives rise to awareness of our body and mind as well as increasing the frequency of positive emotions. This has been shown to increase one's acceptance of pain and increase their pain-pressure threshold.[17] Using yoga to change the internal conversation about pain creates an environment for practitioners to listen to their bodies and decrease pain-related interference (over-thinking, catastrophizing, and preventing one from living their regular lives) while increasing self-efficacy.[18]

The difference between coping and accepting pain was studied by Lance McCracken and Chris Eccleston in 2003. They found that acceptance of pain, as opposed to simply coping with it, decreased the physical limitations their patients were experiencing as well as the anxiety related to the sensations they felt. The study even went so far as to find that those who were able to accept their pain experienced a decrease in the pain itself.[19] Nothing changed in these subjects except their psychological stance towards what they were experiencing. This shows a powerful relationship between the body and the mind, and can be the difference between living a happy life and living one wrought with distress.

In addition to helping with physical pain, yoga practice has also been shown to decrease tobacco use and alcohol consumption, reduce stress, and increase exercise in its practitioners.[20] This has potential to positively affect the community and health care system by decreasing the need for doctor's appointments and hospital visits. There is also good evidence in pregnant women who practice yoga that birth weight increases and pregnancy-induced hypertension is decreased.[21]

The Rise of Injuries in Yoga

Over the last 20 years, yoga injuries have been on the rise and there is growing literature detailing yoga's risks. A 2007 survey conducted of 1336 yoga teachers and yoga therapists from 34 different countries found that poor alignment, previous injury, excess effort, or inadequate instruction were the most common reasons for injury.[22] Tendons, myotendinous junctions (where the muscle and tendon meet), and fibrocartilages such as the spinal discs, menisci in the knee, and labrum in the shoulder and hip are the most likely areas in the body to get injured.[23]

Between 2001 and 2014, there were 29,590 yoga-related injuries seen in United States hospital emergency rooms. Injuries to the trunk accounted for 46.6 percent of the complaints while those to the lower limbs tallied 21.9 percent. The majority of diagnoses were sprain/strain (45%). The overall rate of injury increased from 9.55 per 100,000 in 2001 to 17.01 per 100,000 in 2014.[24] I suspect that number has grown since then.

The same study also found an increase in injury risk based on age category. Students between the ages of 18 and 44 experienced an injury rate of 11.9/100,000 while those between the ages of 45 and 64 a rate of 17.7/100,000. Students 65 and older were the most vulnerable, with a whopping 57.9/100,000 people getting injured. This can easily be explained as a result of the biological changes that take place with aging, such as decreased bone density and sarcopenia (loss of muscle mass, strength, and function that commonly occurs as we get older). Since there was an *increase in overall injury rates* among all age groups, however, factors other than age must be present.

The Canadian Hospitals Injury Reporting and Prevention Program found that 73 percent of yoga-related injuries between 1991 and 2010 occurred after 2005.[25] This provides even more proof that the number of people getting hurt in the practice is dramatically increasing.

One obvious reason for this is that yoga's increased popularity has also demanded a subsequent need for new teachers. The number of newly registered teachers in the US rose by an average of 18 percent from 2008 to 2014. Yoga studios crank out 200-hour teacher training programs (TTPs) several times a year, where typically only 15–20 hours are spent on anatomy and physiology. According to Yoga Alliance, anatomy can also mean teaching esoteric yogic topics such as the chakras (energy centers) and the nadis (energy channels). Thus, a newly trained teacher could graduate from their class with zero education on human biomechanics, kinesiology, muscular anatomy, and injury. This kind of training is nowhere near sufficient to transform a yoga student into a qualified teacher.

Yoga studios are often in a tough bind, though. Many are faced with putting together TTPs or not having enough money to keep their center from going under. Justin Michael Williams, the co-founder of the Business of Yoga consulting firm, says, "Everybody knows if you need to make money, if you need to keep your studio afloat, you do a teacher training."[26] These trainings can bring in anywhere from $2000 to $5000 more per student each year, and thus it would be a poor business model to not lead a TTP. Sadly, however, there is no governing body to assess a new teacher's skill set and ability to teach. Many simply graduate their TTP and are thrown into the workforce way before they have the maturity, education, knowledge, and experience to safely and intelligently conduct a class.

Even the three-year, 500-hour Iyengar Yoga TTP I did more than 15 years ago provided insufficient education in anatomy, physiology, and kinesiology. Teacher trainers, especially in the Iyengar system, are so focused on preparing their students to teach each individual asana, a topic of great depth and importance, that they don't have enough time, or possibly enough understanding themselves, to impart the scientific aspects of anatomy, movement theory, and basic biological stretch responses. Students who realize this deficiency are left needing to search out continuing education that first-year college students can get in their Anatomy and Physiology 101 class.

Lack of teacher education is not the only reason students get hurt, though. Repetitive strain injuries are part of the human experience, and anyone who performs an action repeatedly over time is susceptible to this. Many yogis, including me, have felt for years that as long as we're in alignment, we won't get hurt. This is simply not true.

In her article "Inside my injury: A yoga teacher's journey from pain to depression to healing," Meagan McCrary so vulnerably documents her experience of going from being a super yogi featured in *Yoga Journal*, *OM Yoga*, and *Yoga Magazine* to suffering such debilitating pain in her back and thighs that she needed epidurals just so she could move. After finally being approached by Alexandria Crow, another yoga teacher who had injured herself and completely changed the way she practiced and taught, McCrary realized that she "wasn't the only one whose body hurt—that many yoga teachers had similar injuries, and that mine wasn't due to a lack of proper alignment or strength."[27]

Other teachers and advanced practitioners have come to this realization, too. Former *Yoga Journal* editor Kaitlin Quistgaard wrote after reinjuring her rotator cuff in a yoga class, "I've experienced how yoga can heal but also how yoga can hurt—and I've heard the same from plenty of other yogis."[28]

This truth is exemplified incredibly well in one 12-week randomized trial that showed that yoga was more effective at treating back pain than "usual care." The yoga group even maintained better back function at the three-, six-, and 12-month follow-ups. However, the same group reported a higher incidence of increased pain (12 out of 156) compared to the usual care group (2 out of 157).[29] This shows that yoga can yield both greater benefit and greater detriment to its practitioners.

MYTH BUST #2

YOGA IS A PANACEA FOR YOUR PAIN

Many people look to yoga as an answer to their pain, and many will receive it. Yoga can stretch and strengthen the body in ways many other practices can't. The reduction in pain is predominantly determined by the type of physical ailment they are experiencing, the kind of yoga they practice, and the level of education their instructor has. Someone with spondylolisthesis, a condition where a vertebra has shifted forward, should not do back bends as that puts more pressure on the spine to move forward. Someone with a herniated disc should avoid forward bends as these put more pressure from the disc onto the nerve. These are common spinal conditions that many yoga teachers don't know anything about. Attending a class without a proper understanding of what one is experiencing is a bit like playing Russian roulette. Sometimes you'll get it right and sometimes you won't. This is why when someone with an injury asks me if they should go to a yoga class, we have to have a very detailed discussion before I give an answer.

In 2012, William J. Broad published an article in *The New York Times* called "How yoga can wreck your body."[30] He interviewed my old mentor Glenn Black, who had been vocal for many years about the potential dangers the practice of yoga carried with it. Broad, himself, was a lifelong practitioner with an underlying back issue that he initially found yoga was able to help. But in 2007, doing a relatively innocuous pose—*parsvakonasana* (side flank pose)—his back gave out, shattering his belief that yoga was the panacea for his pain.

Black, himself, after many years of intensive practice, wound up developing severe spinal stenosis (a narrowing of the space between the vertebrae that puts excessive pressure on the nerves) from extreme back bends and twists, and eventually needed a spinal fusion. He had been living in pain for years and was told by doctors that he may eventually lose his ability to walk. The surgery helped relieve a lot of his distress but is hardly the goal he had hoped for from decades of yoga practice.

This did not hinder his love for movement, though. It informed him of more intelligent ways to take care of his body and teach his students. Even before his surgery, he transformed his teaching from traditional asana to remedial joint movements and range-of-motion exercises. He applied science to his teachings rather than blind faith in yoga asana. He became clear that building functional, usable strength is more important than fitting your body into a figure designed by an Indian sage anywhere between 75 and 2500 years ago. He is one of the most influential people in my life and his teachings are sprinkled throughout this book.

Studying the data

The data on yoga injuries can be misleading, though. One study from Gainesville, Florida, showed less than 1 percent of yoga students get injured[31] while a broader study in Australia showed only 2.4 percent of students report getting injured while in class.[32] This is a very small number and hardly of concern compared to the injury rate of sports-related injuries among individuals 25 and over. Cyclists are injured at a rate of 12.6 percent, basketball players 6.12 percent, and baseball 4.13 percent.[33]

The faculty of health science at Sydney University found that 10 percent of the students who practiced at two prominent New York City yoga studios got hurt.[34] Participants here were mostly women and complained of wrist, elbow, and shoulder pain. Because women often have less upper-body strength than men, they also have a higher incidence of shoulder, wrist, and elbow pain in yoga. This is most likely due to the amount of weight bearing on the hands in poses that are repeatedly taught such as down dog, plank and *chaturanga* (4-limbed pose).[35]

Another study at three different Ashtanga yoga centers in Finland showed that 62 percent of the practitioners reported having had at least one injury lasting one month or more. Several of the practitioners expressed having more than one injury. The most common injuries were to the lower back and lower extremities, especially in the hamstrings or knees.[36]

What defines an injury is quite important here, and each of the studies above defined it differently. In Gainesville, Holton and Barry defined a yoga injury as an event that led to lost yoga participation time. In Australia, Penman *et al.* defined it as an event requiring medical treatment or causing prolonged pain, discomfort, suffering, or loss of work. And at the Ashtanga center in Finland, Mikkonen *et al.* defined a yoga injury as a musculoskeletal injury with pain that lasted longer than one month.[37] You'd think the time duration required to qualify as an injury here would decrease the injury rate, but they still found 62 percent of the practitioners reported being hurt. This suggests that Ashtanga yoga's primary and secondary series, which involve practicing many advanced poses in a "pose/counterpose" manner, could create a greater risk of injury than other styles.

For the sake of our own definition, I'll define an injury as follows:

An injury is anything that causes pain, limits range of motion, and decreases musculoskeletal function for longer than three days.

And this is quite a common occurrence in yoga.

In addition to the above-mentioned lack of teacher education and incidence of repetitive stress injuries *any time* an action is repeated over and over, "ego-driven" practice is another major cause of injury. Many yogis, when asked, will take responsibility for their injuries and admit they were "pushing it too far," "trying to look like someone else," or "not listening to their bodies." This is commonly when sprain and strain injuries occur.

This shows us that sometimes it is not the practice of yoga but the *way* we practice that is the issue. It is easy to get caught up in competition, comparison, and striving the same way we do in our regular lives, be it in the workforce, our friendships, or parenting styles. The moment we get fixated on getting somewhere, achieving something we don't already have, or becoming something different, we are in jeopardy of bypassing parts of ourselves and putting our health at risk.

It is important for us, as well, to make a distinction between going to a yoga class and having a private yoga therapy treatment. The latter is a one-on-one situation where a thorough intake is performed and poses/movements are applied specifically for the individual. If the student feels something painful, they are able to communicate that to the therapist. If the therapist sees something that might lead to or exacerbate an injury, they are able to make appropriate and immediate changes. This is simply not possible in group classes where the teacher cannot individually check each student in each pose.

None of this is meant to scare you in any way. The benefits of the practice greatly outweigh its detriments. Like any other form of physical activity, though, yoga carries with it a risk of injury. The way we practice and how deeply we listen to our bodies can determine if we are doing something beneficial or harmful. Exercise is a medicine with a myriad of health benefits, but like any other kind of medication, it must be prescribed properly.

Yoga and Mental Health

Anyone who has taken a yoga class has had the experience of walking in and feeling a certain way, then leaving and feeling completely differently. There is nothing in our external environment that has changed, but what lives inside has shifted. On a chemical level, the body has released oxytocin and other endorphins that change our mood. On a spiritual level, we have taken time to drop everything else going on and attend to what we are feeling. For many of us, that means turning stiffness into mobility and sluggishness into vitality. This makes us feel better and is a large part of why yoga has become a billion-dollar business over the last 20 years. We all want to feel good, and this practice is one way to do it.

Our bodies and minds are connected. Different emotions have an impact on the way we hold and carry ourselves. When we experience shame, grief, or embarrassment, our shoulders roll forward, the chest collapses, and the head lowers. When we experience confidence and charisma, the body is upright and proud.

Yoga practice creates an environment where we are able to access our physical sensations and the mental/emotion states associated with them.

By becoming more intimate with our body through yoga asana, our attitude can change and we are able to shift the way we think and feel about ourselves.

I fell in love with yoga because of its effect not on my body but on my mental health. From a young age, I dealt with insecurity, lack of confidence, and fear. I never felt I was good enough. I grew up as an athlete, and sports gave me a place where I was able to shine. I always felt good on the tennis court or baseball diamond but not really anywhere else.

When yoga came into my life, I found something that combined my natural physical abilities with introspection. I was able to take time every day and do something that brought me an incredible amount of joy but also penetrated the deeper aspects of my psyche. On days I would practice, I felt clear and aligned with my purpose. On days that I didn't, I felt a sense of lethargy and depression.

In recent years, yoga has been the subject of research for its ability to help with stress, depression, addiction, insomnia, schizophrenia, borderline personality disorder, post-traumatic stress disorder (PTSD), attention deficit hyperactivity disorder (ADHD), obsessive compulsive disorder (OCD), and more. Anxiety, which, it could be argued, is a component of all the conditions mentioned above, is known to change breathing patterns, particularly by shortening and speeding up the breath.[38] It has also been shown that anxiety significantly decreases through the practice of yoga, even in college students who attend just one 60-minute class a week.[39]

In 2014, Bessel van der Kolk, author of the definitive book on trauma, *The Body Keeps the Score*, published the first ever research paper on the effects of yoga and PTSD.[40] He found that an eight-week yoga program designed to help sexually abused women had a profoundly greater effect on symptomology than an eight-week program of dialectical behavioral therapy (DBT). He also found that heart rate variability (HRV), which is known to be a sign of regulation between the sympathetic and parasympathetic nervous systems, was balanced through the practice.

HRV is a measure of the variation in the time between each heartbeat. We actually want more variability between heartbeats than less. HRV is controlled by the autonomic nervous system (ANS) which also regulates our blood pressure, breathing, digestion, and other bodily functions that we don't have to think about and that keep us alive. The ANS is subdivided into the sympathetic and parasympathetic nervous systems, which are commonly referred to as the systems that dictate the flight, fight, or freeze responses.

High HRV has a positive impact on our emotional regulation, decision making, and attention capacity. It is often a result of increased parasympathetic activity,[41] which also slows down the heart rate and induces a state of calm.

People with high HRV have been shown to have good cardiovascular fitness and response to stress.

Low HRV is the exact opposite. It is shown in poor decision making, high levels of reactivity, and a decrease in attention span.[42] Low HRV is commonly coupled with a heightened sympathetic nervous system, increased heart rate, and a state of fear or anxiety. It has also been shown to be a factor in various ailments such as cardiovascular disease and liver cirrhosis.

It becomes clear, then, that HRV can be a predictor for different psychological states, and affecting it can have an impact on our moods and relationships. Van der Kolk found that his patients with PTSD had very low HRV and over-responded to minor stresses (a common sign of someone with PTSD) simply because the biological systems that are meant to respond to external stimuli were not up to the task. His research showed that trauma-informed yoga practice raised his patients' HRV and decreased their reactivity.[43]

More recent studies have shown the same, along with the effectiveness of meditation on increasing HRV.[44] Meditation techniques which are aimed at observing our experiences without reacting to them have the effect of calming the mind. We are not trying to stop our thoughts or emotions but simply learning how to recognize and become more intimate with them. This allows us to choose our responses instead of reacting out of habit. This calming of the mind also slows down the heartbeat, increases heart rate variability and shows that there is a direct physiological correlation between the mind and the heart.

Is Yoga Spiritual?

In one of the Buddha's main discourses, the *Sattipathana Sutta* (translated as "the discourse for establishing mindfulness"), he opens by making an unambiguous and profound statement:

> This is the way, monks, for the purification of beings, for the overcoming of sorrow and lamentation, for the destruction of suffering and grief, for reaching the right path, for the attainment of Nibbana, namely, the four foundations of mindfulness.

He then proceeds to list what the four foundations are, the first of these being mindfulness of the body, which he details in great depth. When we understand this—and trust the Buddha's teachings—it becomes difficult to separate the physical asana practice from anything spiritual. Care and attention brought to our bodies is a potential vehicle to freedom from suffering.

The second foundation of mindfulness is called *vedanā*. Vedanā is loosely translated as "feeling tone" or "sensations." It is the bare experience we all have and is divided into three types—pleasant, unpleasant, and neutral. It arises every moment our consciousness comes into contact with an external object or thought. When we eat, have a conversation, watch a movie, brush our teeth, make love, or go for a walk, vedanā is living under the surface. How we consciously or unconsciously respond to it affects how we feel.

The Buddha taught that human beings tend to cling to pleasant sensations, reject unpleasant ones, and space out or lose mindfulness when something is neutral. His teachings focus us to become aware of these experiences, the vedanā, and to develop a sense of equanimity with them. This means not craving for or avoiding anything we feel, while also developing an understanding that everything that arises will also pass away. This is what he called "anicca," or the law of impermanence. He also said that one moment of truly seeing anicca is more valuable than a lifetime of not.

This is also where yoga in the West has failed. There is little instruction on how to direct the mind, mostly because teachers themselves are not taught to do this. Most students in class are comparing, competing, judging, fearing, or over-exerting, instead of developing a keen sense of awareness and understanding about the intricacies of their own human consciousness. Perhaps this level of mindfulness is not actually what asana—in the context of a class—is meant to do, despite the promise imparted by so many teachers over the years. There is a chance that the asana practice's only purpose is to momentarily enliven us and prepare the body to be able to sit for hours on end where true mindfulness can develop. It may be too difficult for the average yoga practitioner to experience an influx of ever-changing sensations while in various poses and still apply effective psychospiritual teachings to their practice. This is also probably why so many advanced yogis eventually turn to meditation at a certain point in their journey. Their deeper spiritual desires have not been fulfilled, and they are willing to let go of what they've known and enter a new terrain to achieve them.

Being in the Body

Many people in today's world "live in their heads" and have forgotten their body even exists. This is often a reaction to a traumatic experience or an increase in stress. When the physical sensations or emotional anguish are greater than the capacity to be present with them, most people "check out" and distance themselves from feeling.

Emotions are an intricate part of self-development and the spiritual path, yet there is very little support for them in the container of a yoga class. Group classes make it difficult for a teacher to pay close attention to the experiences of each student, and, as previously mentioned, most teachers don't have the skill set to guide those in their classes in the psychospiritual realm. This takes truly being a yogi, understanding the mind, and having done a lot of your own inner work. Teachers are also often stretched thin—with low pay, long hours, and insufficient resources. None of this creates a safe environment for deep interpersonal exploration.

While practitioners may experience emotional releases during a class, not many traditions encourage intimacy with this. Iyengar yoga practices mindful, stern, concentrated asanas. This allows practitioners to move above their emotional experience by concentrating their mind. The Bikram practice, which is taught in 105°F (40°C) rooms, is fraught with competition and people bypassing their limits to achieve greater flexibility. The Ashtanga practice moves so quickly from pose to pose that the space to observe what arises is significantly limited.

Yoga brings us into our bodies. There is no questioning that. It's because of this, however, that deeper emotional wounds will also arise; without proper guidance, the student is left stranded, not really understanding what is happening or what to do about it.

The first conscious step in this process is to familiarize yourself with what you are feeling. So many people walk around in reactivity to their experience, not even knowing what's affecting them. Men commonly feel capable of experiencing anger, but when asked what else may be arising, go completely blank. I remember on a meditation retreat in 2005 being asked to observe my emotions and the only one I could come up with for weeks was sadness. It took months of practice to acknowledge joy, happiness, shame, embarrassment, excitement, fear...

The emotions we experience also have correlating physical sensations. Becoming attuned to these physical sensations allows us to cultivate self-awareness without necessarily needing to associate a particular story behind them. Left unchecked and unrecognized, however, these sensations/emotions/feelings dictate our life. A famous quotation, attributed to Carl Jung, says, "Until you make the unconscious conscious, it will rule your life and you will call it fate." Our job with yoga is to explore every aspect of our physical and emotional body, not so we can change it, but so we can understand it. There is a relaxation that comes when we accept and know who we are and release the need to turn into something different. A sense of intimacy with each of our experiences develops and an environment is bred where we can be more responsive and less reactive.

The Psychosomatic Experience

The word "somatic" comes from the Latin word *sōma*, which means body. Somatic means "of or relating to the body." The word "psychosomatic" comes from the Greek and combines sōma with psykhē, or mind. Psychosomatic describes the link between our bodies and minds.

A psychosomatic disorder is a condition where mental and emotional stresses adversely affect the physiological function of the body. This is commonly a result of unprocessed emotional stress or trauma that has led to over-thinking, anxiety, dysfunctional breathing patterns, poor posture, and some sort of physiological or musculoskeletal dysfunction/pain.

Somatic therapy is any form of therapy that incorporates physical and psychological practices into its methods. Yoga and martial arts are probably the first somatic practices known to humans as both aimed at mastery and unification of body and mind. Dance, Pilates, the Feldenkrais method, massage, and intentional breathwork practices are other examples.

Thomas Hanna, a philosophy professor and movement theorist, coined the term "somatics" in the 1970s. He proposed that the experience of physical pain is often a result of "sensory motor amnesia."[45] This is a condition where the neurons in the brain have forgotten how to properly control the actions of the muscles (see the section on motor control later in this chapter). Hanna claimed that through mindfulness and intentional movements akin to physical therapy, a patient can reinvigorate their mind–body pathways and relieve chronic pain.

The places where neural pathways are blocked are areas where the mind and body have lost connection. This can be caused by an acute injury such as a fall but can also develop from traumatic situations or other unprocessed emotions. When there are parts of ourselves that we are hiding from or ashamed of, it will eventually show up in our body.

In the 1970s, Peter Levine developed a form of therapy called Somatic Experiencing (SE). SE is a body-focused approach that concentrates specifically on creating awareness of the inner physical sensations. These sensations are viewed as being the carriers of trauma. "When humans experience trauma," Levine says, "they can become trapped in the freeze part of the flight, fright or freeze response. This stunted development leads to persistent somatic and emotional dysregulation of the nervous system."[46]

In his book *In an Unspoken Voice: How the Body Releases Trauma and Restores Goodness*, Levine says that PTSD symptoms are:

> an expression of stress activation and an incomplete defensive reaction to a traumatic event. The goal of therapy is to release the traumatic activation through an increased tolerance of bodily sensations and related emotions, inviting a discharge process to let the activation dissipate.[47]

Both Levine and van der Kolk have been leading contributors to the therapeutic process of working with PTSD and trauma. They have seen that many mental health conditions have their roots in unprocessed trauma and are not necessarily a death sentence if the person is able to approach their pain with care, compassion, and support. They have also shown that the healing process is a mind and body experience where awareness of our physical sensations and breathing patterns is just as important as therapeutically talking about what ails us.

Emotions show up in our bodies in other ways, too. I have had eight knee surgeries on my right knee as a result of tearing my anterior cruciate ligament (ACL) and meniscus playing ultimate frisbee on July 9th, 2013. It would be so easy to dismiss this as a freak incident and subsequent failed surgeries, but I've never been able to see it that way. My knee has a direct correlation to my sense of self and lack of self-worth. The circumstances that led to the injury entailed me avoiding two different challenging yet potentially nurturing situations, because I was dealing with social anxiety. Had that anxiety not been there, or had I been willing to face it head on, this injury might have never happened. Each surgery has begged me to heal my fractured sense of self, and I'm grateful for where I sit today. I feel better about who I am than I ever have, and I've become a bit of knee expert in the process.

Pain is calling us to something, asking us to bring our attention inwards. Investigating our experience and becoming more intimate with its physical and emotional components can be a rich journey towards wholeness. But there's something that should be made clear: The fact that we are all psychosomatic beings does not give your yoga teacher, physical therapist, or body worker the right to dismiss your back/knee/shoulder pain and say it's an emotional issue. Statements like this invalidate what you're feeling and don't provide an educated path towards healing. Even if there are emotional components to someone's pain that must be addressed, there are also movement patterns associated with it that need to be corrected. One of my clients was told in her initial treatment with a therapist that her hip pain was a result of her menstrual cycle. After working with her just once, I sent her for an MRI scan that revealed a tear in the psoas and the labrum. The therapist had simply made something up because he didn't have the skill set to treat her properly. Had she believed him, she would have gone down a path of thinking there was something wrong with her when really there was a significant physical issue causing her pain.

Techniques for Releasing Emotional Tension

Should you find yourself feeling emotionally stuck in your yoga practice, one ancient yogic technique for moving energy is called the lion's breath. The lion's breath is the only pose within the asana section of Swami Swatmarama's *Hatha Yoga Pradipika* that is not a static pose. The *Pradipika*, or *Light on Yoga*, was written around the 15th century and covers methods far beyond asana, such as breathing techniques, meditations, internal cleansing approaches, concentration techniques, and sexual practices.

To perform the lion's breath, the yogi assumes a seated position, takes a deep breath, and forcefully exhales the air through the mouth while sticking out the tongue and looking upwards with the eyes (Figure 1.1). You can see why this is rarely taught in class—it's hard to accomplish without half of the students cracking up while the other half just feel downright awkward.

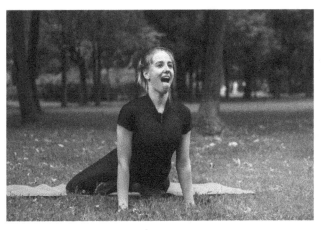

FIGURE 1.1 LION'S BREATH, EYES OPEN

The lion's breath is more of a personal practice than a group experience. It can be used as an emotional release and a way to connect with anger, anxiety, or any other frozen mind state. Keeping the eyes closed instead of open (Figure 1.2) helps connect us with what we are feeling inside. By developing sensitivity to that while performing this technique one is able to observe the changes that take place with the emotions. On a given day, three lion's breaths may clear the cobwebs so you are able to feel free. On another day, it may be ten. The most important aspect of this is listening to your moment-by-moment needs.

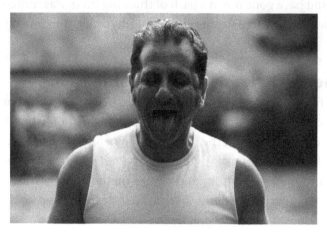

FIGURE I.2 LION'S BREATH, EYES CLOSED

MYTH BUST #3

YOGA WILL HEAL THE DEEPEST PARTS OF YOU

I think it is clear now that yoga, no matter where it's taught or what lineage it's taught in, has spiritual and psychological benefits. I think it's also clear that yoga alone is not a solitary path to healing the depths of your childhood conditioning. There is certainly an overlapping between the spiritual transformation that takes place in a yoga practice and the psychological unraveling that takes place in traditional talk therapy, but when looked at individually, the two are quite different. Yoga can enhance our mood, and that shift of consciousness can be deeply healing, especially over an extended period of time. Just because we are feeling a new sense of aliveness, however, does not mean we have eradicated the root of suffering. We're simply on a good streak. The promise that continued physical practice will eliminate the roots of anger, insecurity, and lack of self-worth is also not true.

One of the biggest mistakes I see (and have made myself) is watching 20-something yogis trying to stretch away their deep-seated emotional tensions and griefs. Our 20s are a time of great development where we can investigate our lives and look at the psychological wounding from our childhood. There is insight that comes from the physical yoga practice, but deep transformation is rarely made if that is the *only* tool we use in our healing.

In addition to our spiritual practices, some form of psychotherapy is also necessary for healing.

The combination of a strong yoga practice accompanied by weekly therapy provides the kind of support we need when facing difficult issues within ourselves. Yoga increases our sensitivity through direct contact with the body and its sensations. Therapy helps to hold the space for whatever may come up as a result. This allows for the body and mind to heal simultaneously.

One of my oldest colleagues, who speaks openly about the emotional distress she experienced in her youth and how she placed so much trust in her asana practice as the vehicle for healing, had to have a hip replacement by her 44th birthday. Her repeated effort to increase flexibility as a means of creating emotional freedom cost her dearly. Her practice and approach to yoga has dramatically changed as a result, and her experience should be a lesson for us all.

If we look at the practice of meditation, we will see how it overlaps with psychotherapy. Both are aimed at the emancipation of suffering and freeing of the mind. However, the two have very different approaches to emotional and physical pain.

Meditation watches the arising and passing of thoughts, feelings, emotions, and mind states. It considers them ephemeral phenomena that come and go. This is especially true of Vipassana in the Mahasi Sayadaw tradition—one of the most widely used meditation techniques and the foundation practice of the Insight Meditation Society in Barre, Massachusetts, and Spirit Rock in Marin County, California. When our attention can see the transient nature of everything we experience, we come closer to understanding anicca, the law of impermanence.

Traditional psychotherapeutic attention, on the other hand, holds on to feelings and turns them over to see what's underneath and how they may relate to something from earlier in life. The experience of anger or insecurity, for example, will be investigated to see when they first arose, why they keep arising now, what the trigger is, how they're affecting our lives, and how we may be able to reprogram ourselves so as to not fall into the same pattern again. Psychotherapy digs, excavates, and stays with the problem until insight is found and the trauma can be released.

Both approaches bring a person into the here and now to become more present. Both bring the person into their body and out of their head, but they are different in how they relate to experience. Psychotherapy is also done in relationship with another person, while even though we may be in a yoga class or mediation retreat with other people, we actually engage in those practices alone.

Jiddhu Krishnamurti, a great Indian philosopher, taught that we know who we are because of our relationships to other people. The Buddha said that *kalyana mitta*, spiritual friends, is one of the most important aspects of the path. Because of this, an important part of our healing must also be in relationship to those around us.

Spiritual Bypassing

In 1984, psychotherapist and Buddhist practitioner John Welwood coined the phrase "spiritual bypassing" to describe a very common pattern he saw: people resorting to spirituality to avoid difficult or painful emotions. He hit the nail right on the head.

Spiritual bypassing uses an aspiration of awakening in an attempt to rise above the unpleasant feelings we may be experiencing. It looks to sneak by the raw and messy aspects of human life and transcend it before we have made peace with it. This is dangerous and can create a difficult split between the enlightened and flawed human we all have within. When we favor certain states of consciousness and reject others, crave particular ways of feeling and avoid others, we create an environment that rejects life's duality instead of cultivating an ease with all of its experiences.

I have seen this very clearly in myself over my years of intense practice. I always told myself I was searching for enlightenment, which actually was true, but at the same time I was simply avoiding the anxiety and fear I woke up with every morning. When I practiced for three to four hours, it would propel me into a state of mind where I was above any of the mental anguish I commonly experienced.

In one of the Buddha's teachings, he espoused that one way to avoid suffering is to develop a state of concentration so deep that the samskaras (latent karmic pains) can't arise. He listed a litany of different techniques to establish this, one of these being a meditation technique called *anapanasati*. *Anapanasati* translates into mindfulness of breath (*sati* means mindfulness and *anapana* refers to inhalation and exhalation). It is a technique where the yogi focuses solely on the sensation of the in and out breath at the base of the nostrils or the rising and falling of the abdomen. When thoughts arise, they are to be discarded, and the attention is immediately brought back to the breath. Instead of investigating the thoughts to understand what's underneath them, they are simply let go. This stills the mind to the point where past and future don't exist, and all that remains is presence.

Anapanasati and the other concentration techniques the Buddha taught were not meant to be the sole practices one used but instead a means for prepping the mind to receive greater insight into the nature of reality. Concentration is a requisite precursor for insight. Since part of the human condition desires the avoidance of suffering, many people who taste the freedom that concentration brings do everything they can to hold on to it for as long as possible. This gripping prevents them from flowing with the vicissitudes and fluctuations of life and keeps them trapped in the cycles of attachment and unhappiness.

Anapanasati, a very powerful and poignant practice, is taught throughout the world and is the base technique used at over 170 meditation centers created by the Burmese master S.N. Goenka. At any ten-day Goenka retreat, the first three and a half days are spent stilling the mind through observing the breath at the base of the nostrils. From there, the practitioner transitions into a Vipassana technique in the Sayadaw U Ba Khin lineage where they mentally scan their body for sensations with the intent of developing equanimity. The entire technique is focused on understanding vedanā and this lays the ground for spiritual insight to manifest.

Spiritual bypassing in our bodies

Spiritual bypassing exists in our bodies, too. As yogis, we often stretch the muscles and joints we're already flexible in, while avoiding the ones we're not. We are literally searching for the places we are already familiar with while circumventing the areas that are unknown. When pain, rigidness, or immobility are felt, they are often avoided due to the amount of attention it demands to truly understand what is needed and what they are saying, both physically and energetically. Exploration of these areas, however, is the exact approach the yogi needs to undertake to free themselves from whatever restriction is being experienced.

Spiritual bypassing in the body probably reveals itself the most in the avoidance of weakness.

One very powerful way to strengthen the hip joint and the muscles around it, which we will go over thoroughly in Chapter 5, is to lie supine, lift one leg into the air with a straight knee and make as wide a circle as you can. While doing this, don't let your opposite hip come off the ground. This isolates your active hip and challenges the motor control of your entire hip flexor complex.

Without fail, there are two or three spots throughout this cycle that everyone struggles with. Go ahead, try it. There are certain points that the psoas and particular fibers of the quadriceps simply don't have control over. What 99 percent of people do in this situation is just avoid those areas and make a smaller version of a hip circle. This is all well and good, but they're skipping over the best part. The weakness is where liberation lies.

To truly strengthen the area and make the complete revolution strong, you have to stop at the exact place of weakness and hold it. By staying there and not "bypassing" it, you are actually creating motor units and sending signals from your brain through your spine into your peripheral muscles. This creates harmony between the mind and the body. It is the true "yoking" that yoga aims to achieve.

Another example would be *virabhadrasana II*. Ideally, the bent leg of this pose makes a 90-degree angle (Figure 1.3). This enables the glute max, quadriceps, knee, and hip joint to all get very strong. But making a 90-degree angle is difficult, so most people stop somewhere around the 60–75-degree range. This is still good and accepted by most teachers, but it does not allow the practitioner to gain the full benefit of the pose. There are still some hurdles and weaker areas to feel to fully gain strength.

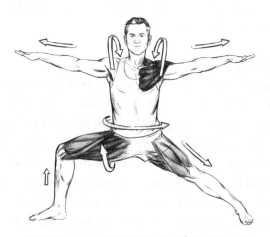

FIGURE 1.3 *VIRABHADRASANA II* (WARRIOR II)

There are many other ways that spiritual bypassing and the emotions we carry live in our bodies. It is far more complicated than many of the new-age books claim. Having back problems does not always equate to feeling unsupported in life or fear of having enough money. A tight psoas does not mean you are having marital problems. But the way we carry and view ourselves in this world does affect our physical bodies, and the path of yoga is one way to explore this.

It is also important for us to differentiate spiritual bypassing from compassion. When there is pain that is too great to deal with—perhaps the sudden loss of a child or spouse—we may need to avoid the depth of those feelings until we have the resolve to face them. This is an act of self-compassion and not spiritual bypassing. Biting off more than we can chew is not courage; it's indiscretion. Compassion is knowing what we can handle and doing it with care. Temporary avoidance of highly intense emotions or sensations can be a wise decision and only becomes spiritual bypassing when we do have the resilience to face them but continue not to.

MYTH BUST #4

WITH PERFECT ALIGNMENT, YOU WILL NOT GET INJURED

I was religiously devoted to Iyengar yoga for more than 15 years. Its slow, methodical approach spoke exactly to the way I liked to inspect my body. Iyengar yoga was a mindfulness practice for me and a way to set my mood for the day. I began the practice for physical reasons but stayed for the psychological benefits that research has shown the practice can bring.

Iyengar yoga's main focus is on alignment, and the physical intention of each pose is to build joint health and tissue integrity. As someone with a background in orthopedic massage and biomechanics, I found Iyengar yoga's approach refreshing. The detail with which Iyengar teachers described each pose showed a level of proficiency I had not seen in any other style.

There is criticism of Iyengar yoga for being purely a physical practice, but I would challenge that to great depths. As the Buddha said in the *Sattipathana Sutta*, the most direct path to liberation is through mindfulness of body. Iyengar yoga's precise focus on specific muscular actions cultivates a deep awareness of our musculoskeletal structure and unites the body and mind. Any practice when done with awareness *is* yoga, and the Iyengar method breeds this. The truth is, the type of asana we are doing is much less important than the presence we bring to our movements, so any type of practice can aid in our personal development. The most spiritual thing in the world can be pointless and the most mundane can be deeply spiritual.

Alignment helps facilitate functional, strong, and healthy joints. It is an important aspect of keeping our bodies healthy. Intuitively, most people know this. When parents tell their kids to sit up straight, there is an innate knowledge that this position is healthier than sitting with collapsed spines and rounded shoulders.

One extraordinary example of the healing potential of joint alignment comes from Glenn Mills, Usain Bolt's running coach. In an interview after Usain broke the world record in the 100m, 200m, and 400m relay, Mills was asked if Bolt had always been this fast and what kind of work he had done with him over the years. He stated that Bolt had always been a superior athlete but also had several injuries as a result of having scoliosis. These injuries were preventing him from becoming the world's fastest man. It was only by hiring a physical therapist to fix the track star's hip, knee, and ankle alignment that he finally overcame his injuries and greatly increased his speed.[48]

Within the yoga world, we've all seen someone in class doing a pose that makes us want to cringe. Their neck is twisted, their spine is contorted, there's clearly too much pressure on the wrong side of their knee. They have not had the proper instruction to safely go into the pose and are attempting to do it the way they think it's supposed to be done. We pray the teacher comes over to save them and focus half our attention the rest of the class on just this. We tell ourselves, "If they keep doing these poses this way, they're going to get hurt."

And they certainly may. Yoga injuries, as we've discussed, are real.

Alignment, however, is not the end-all of movement. Just like anything else in the human body, when done with too much repetition, it can create stress results and wear and tear in the joints. This is basic science and the reason why so many yoga practitioners need hip replacements or have severe arthritis in their 60s.

Around 15 years into my practice, I was in a workshop with my teacher at the time, one of the top Iyengar teachers in the world. He was in his early 60s and mentioned that the doctors told him he needed two shoulder replacements. I had already known he needed two hip replacements, a much more common surgery, but shoulders?! This was a man who had an immaculate asana practice and impeccable alignment. It became clear to me that if I continued to follow the "alignment at all costs" regimen, my path was destined to lead in the same direction. I had already developed an ache in my neck from regular headstands and a bit of pain in my left hip. It was time to make some changes.

Alignment, despite popular belief, does not automatically equate to having functional muscles. As much as people think these two are interchangeable, they are not.

Creating a "bulletproof" body has five main components:

1. alignment
2. flexibility

3. motor control (mobility and strength)
4. variability
5. breath awareness and conscious relaxation.

Alignment describes the optimal position of the joints with a balanced muscular force around them. We can think of alignment in terms of a ball being suspended in the air by a sequence of rubber bands. If all those rubber bands (muscles) are in harmony with one another, the ball (joint) will be right in the center. If a couple of those rubber bands are tighter or looser than others, the ball will be pulled in various directions and will create imbalance. This is the definition of compensation.

Flexibility is defined as the ability to move or bend without breaking. As we've discussed, it's nice to be flexible, but that does not mean we are without pain or discomfort.

Motor control is the brain's ability to control movement by sending signals through the spinal cord into the peripheral muscles.

Voluntary muscle contractions occur when a motor neuron sends a message from the brain and initiates a reactive impulse into motion. Each motor neuron is responsible for exciting a given number of muscle fibers. The muscle fiber and the motor neuron associated with it are collectively called a motor unit. The force of a muscle's contraction is controlled by the number of activated motor units.

It is important for us to understand the difference between a muscle and a muscle fiber. There are around 650 skeletal muscles in the body. In the biceps brachii alone, there are 580,000 muscle fibers.[49] Within the entire body there are tens of millions.

Motor units are classified as either slow twitch or fast twitch. Slow-twitch units are responsible for movements that involve long muscular contractions such as maintaining one's posture. The back muscles multifidus and erector spinae are two examples. Many yoga asanas help to generate strength in these areas.

Fast-twitch units can be broken up into two types; fast fatigable (FF) and fast resistant fatigable (FR). Fast-twitch fibers have less endurance than their counterparts and are responsible for actions that require explosive exertions such as running or jumping. FF examples include the muscles of the eyes, which need to move quickly but for short periods of time. The FR units are more resistant to fatigue than the FF but still produce about twice the amount of force as a slow-twitch unit. The gastrocnemius in the calf is an example of this.[50]

When humans first learn movement patterns, the brain chooses particular combinations and sequences of fibers to activate. These are called motor programs. Those same fibers will be activated over and over again to reinforce and ingrain the specific fiber recruitment pattern. If it's successful, that's great. If the movement we are repeating involves compensation, however, dysfunction and pain will eventually arise.

After an injury, motor control automatically depletes, and part of the healing process involves retraining its capacity. A perfect example of this is something called "quad lag" after an ACL surgery. The body recognizes the surgery as a trauma, and because of the drilling that takes place in the bone, there is a significant amount of inflammation that occurs. One day after surgery, when the nerve block has worn off, there is an inability to engage the quadricep. The first ten days after the surgery are spent simply resting, gently flexing and extending the knee, while regaining (motor) control of the quadricep.

Developing functional motor control is a way to create strength through all the ranges of motion you have available. Where there is flexibility without mobility, we are looser than we are strong. This combination is a breeding ground for injury.

The key to developing motor control is threefold:

1. the mind's present-moment connection with the action taking place
2. the duration and force with which the action is performed
3. the ability to maintain awareness of the breath while keeping the nervous system calm.

Repetitions of an exercise can build strength but can also be done quite mindlessly. Holding a particular movement for extended periods of time, especially in an area of weakness, requires the mind and body to be connected. This creates the cellular system to increase the amount of motor units within the muscle. If load is placed on the muscle being used, more motor units can be recruited. The development of motor units, combined with awareness, increases functional motor control in that specific area.

Maintaining awareness of the breath while keeping the nervous system calm can be difficult and takes focus. The term "conscious relaxation" was first described to me by Glenn Black. It is that place of finding balance between calmness and effort and is something we must apply in our movement and asana practices.

If the breath is not able to be calm, it is time to stop the exercise/asana and return to normal breathing. This brings the body back to homeostasis. This allows us to use the breath as a medium for uniting the body and the mind. The breath is the guru which we follow, while the exercises/asanas are the students learning to become stronger and smarter.

NeuroKinetic Therapy® and Detecting Compensation

NeuroKinetic Therapy is a system of body work that uses manual muscle testing to access the motor control capability of a muscle. The muscle test triggers a response in the motor control center (MCC) of the brain. When a muscle can't complete the task it's being asked to do, the MCC opens itself up for learning.

NKT® can then assess if that muscle is not functioning properly because another muscle in the body is overworking. It is a way of detecting if some areas are neurologically underactive while others are overactive. This is the definition of compensation.

When I found NKT, I was at a crossroads in my body work practice. After six years as a sports massage therapist treating players on the professional tennis circuit, I was bored with my career and approach to the body. NKT offered me a completely different skill set for treating pain, one that revolved around the creation of strength as opposed to solely the release of tightness.

Since 2016, I have been leading NKT classes worldwide, including creating several adjunct yoga and movement-based programs.

One of my favorite examples of compensation came during a class I was teaching in Florida. One of the students presented with a terrible and constant back pain. He was a 25-year-old bodybuilder and was built like a truck. He mentioned he could bench press 375 pounds and squat somewhere around 450.

When asked to pass a simple abdominal motor control test, however, he failed miserably. He also failed the tests for the psoas, erector spinae, gluteus maximus, and multifidus. These are all muscles he had "built" while weightlifting.

As a weightlifter, he was constantly holding his breath and clenching his jaw when he lifted. As a result, his muscles were only functional when he held his breath and clenched his jaw. He had trained his nervous and musculoskeletal systems to live with this dysfunction. This combination caused him to regularly be compressing his facet joints, have neurologically underactive back muscles, and be in constant pain.

Holding the breath and gripping the jaw does actually help someone lift more weight. In NKT, we call these two areas—the diaphragm and masseter— global facilitators. They have the ability to compensate for any muscle in the entire body. But this is no way to live, and it clearly becomes a breeding ground for pain. I would never ask a weightlifter to change their methods as this could be detrimental to their career. I would, however, ask them to perform a 5–10-minute breathing and muscular activation practice before and after they lift. This will help offset the neurological imbalances they are creating while training.

Variability is defined as the normal variations that occur in motor performance across multiple repetitions of a task.[51] Without variability, our movements would be rigid and robotic. Teaching your body to move seamlessly though the ranges of motion it experiences decreases the chance of it being subjected to loads it can't handle. If we were to train our bodies to only be in perfect alignment all the time, the moment we are unintentionally not in that alignment, our tissues would be too fragile to handle the change and injury would occur.

We can see variability in everything we do because when a person tries to repeat the same action twice, it is never exactly the same. If one were to electronically study Tiger Woods swinging a golf club, Tom Brady throwing a football, Lebron James shooting a basketball, Rafael Nadal hitting a tennis ball, or Yo-Yo Ma playing the cello, they would find variations in each action performed. They are all masters of their craft and still vary in their actions. It is for this reason that, in 1967, Bernstein used the expression "repetition without repetition." In this, he describes the uniqueness and non-repetitive nature of motor patterns.[52]

Variability decreases with skill acquisition in one context and increases in another. The difference between Rafael Nadal's forehand and yours or mine is simply his ability to repeat the same motor pattern at a higher frequency. Thus, the variability in his swing has decreased. In the other sense, he's hit so many hundreds of thousands of forehands and has a greater array of variability to his swing that he is able to conduct many different patterns and still produce the desired effect. Thus, he has more variability to his forehand than you or I have.

With our yoga practice, it is crucial to be able to place our joints into alignment, but it is possibly more important to be able to withstand the demands of spontaneous, unexpected movements. Thus, intentionally training patterns out of perfect alignment may be just as important as attaining it. Developing strength in one plane is great. Developing tissue resilience in all planes allows the body to move freely with less risk.

Take, for example, a basketball player who continually sprains their ankle. Most commonly, the ankle rolls and the lateral (outside) ligaments get over-stretched. The load they are being asked to withstand is greater than their capacity to do so. But if that same player had been training their ankle in a controlled, rolled-out position similar to that of the position they sprained it in, their tissue resilience would be greater and the likelihood of an injury would be less. They certainly would have been "out of alignment" during the training process, but their ligaments would have been taught to withstand a certain pressure and position they may accidentally fall into. This would mean they were training their ankle ligaments to experience more variability, which could have reduced the intensity of the injury or prevented it altogether.

In many ways, we can look at this from a psychological perspective, too. Most of us, me included, like to be in control of everything around us. It's an attempt to create safety in an uncertain world. We do everything we can to manipulate our surroundings so we can experience what we want. Yes, this is the root of suffering, but it's difficult to escape. The question then becomes "What if we make our minds and hearts so big that they can handle anything that comes their way?" This would create emotional variability and an ability to adapt to all conditions. This is easier said than done, but it does provide the groundwork for real peace. Now, what if we trained our bodies the same way?

Breath awareness grounds us into the present moment. It is the link between living life in the head and living it in the body. **Conscious relaxation** details an intentional effort to maintain ease in the body when performing a physical task. Many of us walk around tense and anxious in our everyday lives. Even in a yoga class, students will overly force themselves in an effort to go deeper into a pose. This tension is antithetical to what we are attempting to do with our yoga practice.

Properly synchronized breathing, a topic we will discuss in depth in Chapter 3, improves the ventilation of the lungs by increasing the respiratory volume. Increased respiratory volume increases the level of oxygenation of the blood. Increased oxygen to the blood reduces the rate of fatigue in the muscles whereas decreased oxygen supply increases fatigue.[53] Maintaining awareness of the breath will thus significantly aid in achieving the overall effects of exercise.

Awareness of the breath combined with conscious relaxation also helps us to determine where our neural edge is. The neural edge is the place within the nervous system where maximum effort and ease meet. When we find this place, the body is challenged to progress without being overly stressed and subjected to injury. When the neural edge is bypassed, the risk of damaging the tissue is greatened. A weightlifter trying to squat 50 pounds more than they are able to may blow out their knees or back. A yogi trying to do a full split when they can't touch their toes will most likely tear their hamstrings.

Being sensitive to the neural edge means listening to our bodies. It is easier than you may realize to practice yoga and create tension. When tension starts to arise and we begin to exceed our capabilities, it's our responsibility to stop and ensure that we are not compensating or doing harm. Even when performing the sequences in this book, it is your job to listen to what is right for you. If any of the poses or movements are challenging, that is good! If they are taxing on your body in a way that causes your muscles and nervous system to tense and the breath to not flow, that is not good. It is up to you to develop self-agency and sensitivity to your body's capacity, limits, and neural edge.

Understanding the neural edge also allows us to apply the yogic principle of *asteya*—non-theft—to our practice. We can try to "steal" a pose by pushing ourselves too far. We can also shy away from our real capacity and believe we are not as strong or flexible as we are. Both of these are mechanisms that humans, for one reason or another, implement to avoid truly facing themselves. Becoming sensitive to the neural edge and understanding its importance creates a "meet and greet" ground where understanding and change can be made.

CHAPTER 2

Principles of Sports Conditioning

There are four main principles of sports conditioning used by trainers worldwide. These are integrated approaches to ensuring an athlete is as fit and prepared as possible for their sport.

These principles can easily be applied to our yoga therapy practice, as well. Understanding the science of movement and blending the research of the West with the practices of the East creates a more thorough system of healing.

The four principles are:

1. individuality
2. specificity
3. progression
4. overload.

Individuality is something we know quite well as yogis. Our bodies are unique and our capacities vary. In a single yoga class, you can have one person with their foot behind their head and another who can't touch their toes.

Individuality permeates into all aspects of our life. A well-trained psychotherapist knows that the technique they successfully implemented with one patient may not work with another. Their job is to sensitize themselves to the needs of the person in front of them and act accordingly.

Ajaan Chah, a great Buddhist monk, was once criticized for giving two students very different directions. He responded by stating that if he gave the second student the same instruction as he gave the first, it would have been like telling him to walk straight ahead into a ditch.[1]

Understanding where our individual ranges of motion limitations are sets the foundation for where we need to effect change. Knowing exactly where we have weakness allows us to target the area and create strength. Time and time again, injured people are given basic, cookie-cutter exercises by their physical therapists without a proper or accurate assessment. To give a rotator cuff patient the most common rotator cuff exercise—side-lying external rotation strengthening to target the infraspinatus (Figure 2.1)—when they have a minor subscapularis tear (an internal rotator of the glenohumeral joint) could be a waste of time at best and significantly hinder their rehabilitation at worst. We must be accurate in assessing the patient before us to know the right exercises to give.

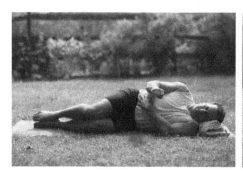 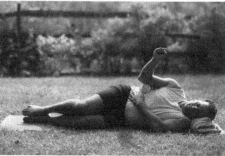

FIGURE 2.1 SIDE-LYING EXTERNAL ROTATION STRENGTHENING TO TARGET THE INFRASPINATUS

Someone who presents with spondylolisthesis—a condition where one of the spinal vertebrae has shifted forward—should not be doing back bends since these put extra stress on the already anterior vertebrae. Back bends, though, are the most frequently indicated exercise for herniated discs. And even people who have herniated discs will vary in which back bends will work for them. *Bhujangasana* (cobra pose) may be perfect for some while *salabhasana* (locust pose) and *setu bhandasana* (bridge pose) will be better for others. Assessment, effect, and individuality are key.

Specificity states that we get better at a particular movement, exercise, or yoga pose the more we practice it. The body adapts in its physical fitness specific to the type of training we are performing. Particular muscle fibers are activated only when those muscles are trained. Playing tennis and practicing your forehand is a great way to improve your tennis skills but a horrible approach to hitting three-pointers in a basketball game.

Training of particular muscle fibers allows for those fibers to be more easily recruited the next time we need them. Over time, muscle memory will develop for these movements so they can be performed without the necessity of direct, intent focus.

The law of specificity blends perfectly with the law of individuality and is particularly important when it comes to therapy. If someone presents with neck pain and the C1–C2 vertebrae are stuck, this is often coupled with difficulty rotating the head to one side. To affect this, they must work on turning their head in this exact motion in order to heal. Other factors may be involved but the individual will not have full cervical rotation by simply practicing neck flexion.

This does not mean, however, that we must only practice the one movement we find difficult in order to improve. Tennis coaches give very specific tennis-related drills for their players, but doing box jumps, something that is certainly not tennis specific, can strengthen the legs and produce more force during a serve. A yogi who wants to get into full *urdvha dhanurasana* (wheel pose), can practice bridge poses as a preparatory phase for warming up pelvic mobility. They can even practice *urdvha hastasana* (hands-in-the-air pose) or *gomukhasana* (cow face pose) as a way to prepare the shoulders. The law of specificity thus allows similarities between training and goal performances.

The primary goal of specificity training is to condition the muscles and the joints that will be used in the target activity. Once achieved properly, repetition then reinforces the fiber recruitment pattern. In the example of turning the neck to one side, the splenius capitis, anterior scalene, sternocleidomastoid, and rectus capitis must all work in sync with one another. If they do not, the body compensates and discomfort ensues. If they do, it harmonizes, and we should repeat the action over and over again to ingrain the fiber recruitment pattern more effectively. When our ranges of motion, motor control, and strength goals are complete, we are often healed from the pain that was previously ailing us.

Progression details the need to increase our workload the more the body is capable of successfully performing the task at hand. If we are aiming for improvements in range of motion or strength, the practices we are performing must be regularly altered so that the body is forced to adapt to the changing and more challenging stimuli.

Progression becomes vitally important in therapy. The external rotation exercise that is commonly given to rotator cuff patients that we spoke about earlier may be very difficult to do for someone with an infraspinatus tear. They may only be able to do this exercise with zero weight for the first week. The goal would be to simply restore some of the motion itself. After a week of repetition, they may be able to add a little resistance and perform the exercise using a band. And after, that they may progress to using a one-pound weight, then two pounds, and so forth. We constantly have to assess the gains that are made and move our clients appropriately.

If we wanted to increase our hamstring flexibility, for example, we can start with *supta padangusthasana* (reclining hand-to-big-toe pose), a simple supine one-legged hamstring stretch. After a week of doing this, however, our tissues will adapt and the gains we were making may plateau. To continue to progress, we'll have to challenge the hamstrings through different asanas and on different planes.

The progression principle basically says that in order to progress, we need to put additional stress on our body by increasing three things: frequency, intensity, and time.

- **Frequency** refers to the number of times we perform an exercise. If we were practicing that initial hamstring stretch once a day and it became easy, we can increase the frequency to twice a day.
- **Intensity** refers to how hard we are training in a particular exercise. If we are stretching our hamstring to 90° the first week, we can see if it's safe now to push it to 95° or 100°.
- **Time** refers to how long we are doing the exercises for. If we started at 60 seconds, we can progress to 75 and so forth.

Overload and progression are very similar, just like individuality and specificity are. In fact, some people combine the two and use the phrase "progressive overload." Progressive overload describes the gradual increase of stress needed to be placed on the body for continued improvement. Since the body's adaptive capabilities will only respond if required to exert a greater magnitude of force to meet higher physiological demands, without progressive overload, we will plateau.

Plateauing may be perfectly fine in the case of working with an injury once it is healed. The client may not have a desire for greater gains since the goal was simply to regain function and remove pain. But in order to continue to progress and increase muscular hypertrophy (increased muscle mass as a result of exercise), overload is critical.

There are several ways to increase overload but the two that I am concerned with for the sake of this book are:

- increased load
- increased repetitions.

In regard to load, this means increased weight added to whatever we are doing. Since we will not be adding any external weight in the sequences included in

PRINCIPLES OF SPORTS CONDITIONING   49

this book, I am referring to what is known as weight bearing. Weight bearing is the percentage of weight placed on a particular joint. Standing puts weight on the ankles, knees, hips, and spine. It is a way of increasing load on the joints compared with lying down. Plank pose, for example, muscularly loads the triceps, wrist extensors, abdominals, and quadriceps. *Utkatasana* (chair pose), which we will use in Chapter 4, primarily loads the erector spinae, multifidus, quads, and glutes. To increase the load in either of these, we can increase the time we hold them for. In *utkatasana*, we can deepen our squat to put more stress on the ankles, knees, hips, quads, and glutes. If we wanted to increase repetitions once we become more proficient, we may decide to do five sets instead of three.

This concept of overload is possibly where the phrase "it's got to hurt if it's to heal" came from. There is wisdom in this because it states that we must challenge the body in order for it to adapt to more functional capabilities. There is also a lot of misinformation inferred from the phrase because pain, especially when working out, getting a massage, or doing a yoga practice, is not always a good thing. We do not have to hurt to heal. There are good pains and bad pains, and we must use our intuition and intelligence to determine which is which.

We also never want to unconsciously increase load. This can, and often does, lead to injury. Small increments in the 2.5–5 percent range normally lead to gains and increased capacity.

Types of Muscles

There are three types of muscles: skeletal, cardiac, and smooth.

Skeletal muscles attach to our bones and are responsible for all voluntary movements. Cardiac muscle pumps blood from the heart. Smooth muscle is responsible for involuntary movements, such as in the stomach and intestines where it helps with digestion, or the urinary system where it functions to rid the body of toxins.

Skeletal and cardiac muscles are both known as striated muscles because they appear with long, parallel stripes. Skeletal muscles are composed of muscle fibers, and those fibers contain something called myofibrils. Within each myofibril is something called a sarcomere. A sarcomere is the basic contractile unit of a muscle. The sarcomere contains filaments called actin and myosin. Myosin is a thick filament, whereas actin is thin. When these two filaments slide past each other, the sarcomere shortens and the muscle contracts. This contraction transmits itself through the muscle and tendon to the bone, thus creating movement.

Excessive sarcomere strain is the primary cause of injury. The inflammation that occurs after injury will further degrade the tissue, but prevention of the inflammation, which we will discuss later, leads to a possible long-term loss in muscle function.[2]

Types of Muscular Contractions

There are three types of muscular contractions: concentric, eccentric, and isometric.

Concentric contractions produce muscle shortening. Since muscles act and bones move, when a concentric contraction takes place, the angle of the joint becomes smaller. When someone flexes their elbow to show how big their muscles are, the biceps brachii muscle shortens while the elbow joint anteriorly compresses.

Eccentric contractions take place when a muscle lengthens while it contracts. This occurs when the force applied to the muscle exceeds the force produced by the muscle itself. When doing a bicep curl with weight similar to what we just described, the action of straightening the arm causes the biceps brachii to lengthen while it is still contracting. Another example of this would be lowering the torso after an abdominal crunch. The abs are still contracting but they are lengthening at the same time. Skeletal muscles are also eccentrically contracting to support our body weight against the force of gravity.

Eccentric contractions, when compared to concentric or isometric, produce a greater force while requiring less oxygen and energy.[3] The metabolic cost required for eccentric exercise is approximately four times lower than the same exercise performed concentrically.[4] Because of this, eccentric training is recommended for those with age-related sarcopenia and neurological and musculoskeletal diseases because they are easier to perform.[5]

Eccentric contractions, however, also cause more tissue damage than their counterparts. When uncontrolled, this is what commonly causes a muscle strain. When controlled and intentional, the tearing that takes place in the sarcomeres increases the rate of satellite cell, fibroblast, neutrophil, and macrophage production to the injured muscle tissue. These cells increase waste removal and speed up the healing capacity of the tissue.[6] This is why eccentric contraction is also a commonly used technique in the rehabilitation of tendinopathies and other sports-related injuries.[7]

Isometric contraction describes a sustained contraction against an immovable force that produces no change in length of the involved muscle group. If one attempted a bicep curl with a weight that was greater than their capacity to lift it, they would be performing an isometric contraction for the biceps brachii. Another example of an isometric hold is plank pose. With the arms outstretched, the legs fixed, and the abdomen engaged, this is a full-body isometric contraction for the triceps, quadriceps, and abdominals. (In August 2021, Daniel Scali of Australia broke the world record for the longest plank pose ever held, at nine hours and 30 minutes. Try holding it for one minute and let me know how it goes.)

Isometrics are particularly attractive after an injury because they are performed with minimal movement to the joint and thus reduce the risk of exacerbating the injury. Since concentric contraction and eccentric contraction produce a shearing effect on joints, isometrics can be optimally used to reduce muscle atrophy and aid in promoting the recovery process.[8]

There is ample research that points to isometrics being the most effective type of contraction in regard to tissue healing. They create maximal recruitment of muscle fibers without causing wear and tear.[9] Bone density, tendons, muscles, ligaments, and joint capsules all get stronger. Isometric contractions also don't increase inflammatory cells,[10] so they are able to be practiced without creating more harm.

When using isometrics to heal a tendon injury, Oranchuk *et al.* found that a force of at least 70 percent of maximum voluntary contraction is required.[11] The length of the individual isometric hold, however, does not appear to be as significant in terms of pain reduction as the total duration of time practiced. Short-duration (24 sets of 10 seconds, 240 seconds total) and long-duration (six sets of 40 seconds, also 240 seconds) loading isometric knee extension at 85 percent voluntary contraction for four weeks both produced significant pain relief in a patellar-loading single-leg decline squat, also known as a pistol squat.[12]

Long-duration holds, however, have been shown to increase stiffness of the tendinous structures when compared to shorter-duration contractions. Thus, if one is repairing a damaged tendon and attempting to reduce its elasticity, longer holds are recommended.[13]

Muscle Strains

Muscle strains are commonly referred to as pulled muscles. A strain occurs when the load placed on the muscle is greater than its capacity to withstand the load. Muscles often tear during the eccentric phase of contraction—that is, when they're lengthening and contracting at the same time. They are presented with an immediate and sudden onset of localized pain.

Strains frequently occur in muscles that cross two joints, because these muscle have a greater contraction velocity and a greater capacity to change length but less capacity to withstand tension.[14] Examples of these muscles are the rectus femoris (anterior hip and knee), biceps femoris (posterior hip and knee), and the gastrocnemius (posterior knee and ankle). Muscle strains can occur in three different locations: within the muscle itself, at the musculotendinous junction, or at the osteotendinous junction where the tendon attaches to the bone.

There are three grades of muscle and tendon strains:

- **Grade 1:** Minimal damage to the individual muscle fibers (less than 5%). This is coupled with minimal loss of strength and range of motion. These tears can take anywhere from one to four weeks to heal.
- **Grade 2:** More extensive damage and more muscle fibers are torn. There is a significant loss of strength and function in addition to possible bruising and swelling. These tears generally take 6–12 weeks to fully heal.
- **Grade 3:** This is a complete rupture to the muscle or tendon. Pain is severe and surgery is often required to reattach the damaged muscle or tendon.

Tendon Injuries

Muscles connect to tendons, and tendons connect to bones. The attachment area of the muscle to the tendon is called a musculotendinous or myotendinous junction. The attachment of a tendon to a bone is called the osteotendinous junction. There is less blood supply to tendons than to muscles, and thus the healing process is longer due to the decrease in vascularization.

In the United States, more than 33 million musculoskeletal injuries are reported each year. Fifty percent of those involve tendon and ligament injuries.[15] Tendon injuries do not only occur in athletes and physically active adults but also appear in the sedentary population after moderate activity.[16] Tendinopathies such as tendinitis are microtears that create inflammation of the tendon and are often accompanied by pain. Tendinosis is a degenerative condition within the tendon and does not present with evidence of an inflammatory response.[17]

The remodeling process of the tendon has been shown to be positively impacted by implementing load to the injured tissue. This can include gradual return to activity as well as various strength training techniques. Rest, however, as we will describe shortly, has actually been shown to slow down the recovery process.

Ligaments sprains are tears to the ligament and can be categorized in the same way as strains. Ligaments, however, have less blood supply than tendons or muscles and thus the healing process takes longer. A grade 2 sprain will take 2–3 months and grade 3 will require surgery.

The most famous type of grade 3 ligament tear, or full ligament rupture, is an ACL tear. There are between 100,000 and 200,000 ACL tears a year in United States which translates into one out of every 3500 Americans.

The RICE Myth

In 1978, Dr. Gabe Mirkin coined the term RICE in his best-selling book, *The Sports Medicine Book*.[18] RICE stands for rest, ice, compression, and elevation. It was believed this was the most effective approach to treating acute injury.

His statements in the book were predicated on outdated research from nearly four decades ago, and in 2015, Mirkin himself recanted these beliefs and admitted his error.

Recent research has actually shown that rest and ice can delay recovery. "Gentle movement helps tissues heal faster and the application of cold suppresses the immune responses that start recovery," says Gary Reinl is his book *Iced! The Illusionary Treatment Option*,[19] for which Mirkin wrote one of the forewords.

After an injury, there are three phases of healing that must sequentially occur for the muscular tissues to return to health.[20] They are:

1. degeneration/inflammation
2. repair/regeneration
3. remodeling.

Degeneration is characterized by rupture and necrosis (death) of the myofibers. A hematoma/bruise is often formed and scar tissue develops.

Inflammation is the body's natural defense response, governed by the immune system. It occurs when the body is impacted by an irritant. This could be a germ, a torn muscle, a bruise, or even a splinter. When this impact occurs, the body sends white blood cells to the site of injury to protect it from infection. This often causes the redness and swelling associated with inflammation.

Inflammation must successfully occur in order for the body to shift its focus to the repair/regeneration phase. The repair/regeneration phase must also then be completed before proceeding to the remodeling phase.

Inflammation that is produced after an injury is done uses the same biological mechanisms that are used to kill germs. Inflammatory cells, called macrophages, release a hormone called insulin-like growth factor (IGF-1) into the damaged tissues, which helps the muscles heal. Applying ice to reduce this inflammation delays the healing by preventing the body from releasing IGF-1.

Inflammation is thus clearly the first phase of healing and not an undesired outcome that needs to be reduced or delayed. It is an instantaneous protective mechanism with the primary objective of controlling the extent of cell injury and preparing the tissue for the process of repair.[21] Although inflammation further degrades the tissue, prevention of inflammation leads to long-term loss in muscle function.[22]

That is not to say ice is useless and doesn't reduce pain. It is often used as a short-term analgesic since it numbs the tissue and can decrease sensation. If that is the goal, then ice can be effective. The practitioner should be aware, however, that this will not positively affect the long-term outcome, and it has also been shown to temporarily reduce strength, speed, endurance, and coordination.

The **repair/regeneration** phase usually starts within 3–4 days after the injury. Blood supply to the injured skeletal muscle begins to occur and is essential for successful healing. This revascularization process prevents a deepening of the fibrosis, or a thickening and scarring of the connective tissue.[23]

The regeneration of the torn myofibrils is done by something called a satellite cell. Satellite cells are precursors to skeletal muscle cells. During embryonic development, satellite cells are stored below the basal lamina of each myofibril. When a lesion occurs to a muscle, these once-latent cells proliferate and spread into the myofibrils and differentiate into myoblasts. Myoblasts are the precursor cells that form new muscle fibers.[24] There is also evidence suggesting that satellite cells are capable of fusing with existing myofibers to facilitate growth and repair.[25]

The **remodeling phase** includes maturation of the newly regenerated myofibers. This creates recovery of the muscle's functional capacity. When the once-injured myofibers are reinnervated by the nerves, and the synaptic contact between them and the motor neuron has taken place, the remodeling phase is complete.[26]

So if RICE is not the path, what is?

There is an abundance of research that suggests moving early in the recovery process is more beneficial than extended periods of rest. Many new acronyms have been recommended, but there are two that I enjoy the most and ascribe to in my therapy treatments.

The first is from Reinl, who proposed ARITA, which stands for "active recovery is the answer." Active recovery can be any movement that includes contraction of skeletal muscle that was previously subjected to trauma.[27] The key to active recovery is to ensure that the movements being practiced remain pain-free. Reinforcing a pain signal to the brain over and over again can trick it into thinking it's still in trouble when it's not.

In 1999, Buckwalter and Grodinsky promoted the value of placing a load on damaged tissues to enhance the recovery process. They stated that "although new approaches to facilitate bone and fibrous tissue healing have shown promise, none has been proven to offer beneficial effects comparable to those produced by loading healing tissues."[28]

In a 2016 study on the effects of muscular activation after extreme exertion, it was concluded that 20 minutes of active recovery using the same muscles that were stressed during exercise is more effective in fatigue reduction than using muscles that weren't previously being used.[29]

> The recovery can likely be attributed to the fact that contraction of the tissues previously subjected to trauma enhances blood circulation and lymphatic drainage, which facilitates the successful evacuation of metabolic waste products from the affected area. As a result, the process of inflammation can be completed, and the next two phases of recovery (repair and remodeling) can begin.[30]

The other acronym that effectively describes a treatment plan and moves us away from RICE is MEAT. MEAT stands for movement, exercise, analgesia, and treatment.

Movement and exercise take a damaged area through pain-free ranges of motion and help push inflammation through the body and increase the speed of the repair phase of healing. Movement immediately after an injury also decreases our fear around what we are experiencing. By making pain-free contact with the injured tissue, a signal is sent to our brain that we can do something about the injury. This takes courage since our instincts often tell us that movement is a potential threat and can cause more harm.

Analgesia is the inability to feel pain. When we are in too much pain, it limits our ability to move. Ice is an analgesic, as are nonsteroidal anti-inflammatory drugs (NSAIDS) such as ibuprofen and naproxen. NSAIDs inhibit the synthesis of prostaglandins which initiate inflammation,[31] so the practitioner should know that they are solely attempting to reduce pain, and the healing process may be delayed as a result. However, as we discussed earlier, when the pain is too great, doing something about it is a form of compassion, not distraction.

Treatment is a topic we have not yet discussed at great length outside the realm of movement and yoga therapy. Treatment can be any hands-on technique performed by a skilled practitioner. Massage therapy, chiropractic, and acupuncture are three of the most common forms. Massage has been proven to help restore damaged tissue and is known to be the most effective technique for reducing delayed onset muscle soreness (DOMS).[32] Massage also increases blood flow to the muscles and helps push lymph through the body, thus aiding in the healing process. In addition, it is able to break up scar tissue and speed up muscle recovery.[33]

When muscles get tight, the connective tissue and fascicles that form the muscles lose their glide. This creates trigger points. A trigger point is an area within a muscle that has become rigid and dense. It is often painful and presents with greater sensitivity and abnormal texture when palpated by a therapist. A skilled therapist will be able to feel into your tissue and know which areas are tight and which are not, just as a computer technician can determine where the glitch is in your system. There is also often a twitch response within the muscle when the trigger point is touched. Common trigger point locations are in the rhomboids, upper trapezius, quadratus lumborum, gluteus medius, biceps femoris, and gastrocnemius, among others.

Although a particular type of stretching called post-isometric relaxation has been proven to reduce as much as 94 percent of the pain associated with trigger points, a lasting effect on point tenderness has only been observed in 23 percent of these people.[34] With this information, it becomes even more important to include massage of the trigger points to reduce pain and recover from injury. Trigger point injections and dry needling have also become more popular and are now being prescribed by doctors and performed in hospitals.

The calming effect of massage therapy, acupuncture, or even chiropractic treatments on the nervous system should not be underestimated, either. When our body is tense, it is more difficult for us to heal. Creating a state of physical and emotional relaxation can greatly aid in the process of returning us back to normal.

Good Pain vs. Bad Pain

As we've discussed, human beings generally tend to avoid pain at all costs. We want to feel pleasure, not the opposite. This spans the entire range of existence, including its physical, emotional, psychological, and spiritual aspects.

This is also why our suffering perpetuates. The Buddha taught that there is suffering in life and that the way to relinquish it is not through avoidance but through fully meeting our experience and not wishing for anything to be different.

Intellectually, most of us understand this. Experientially, most of us reject our unpleasant experiences and suffer.

When working with pain, the first question we should ask is: "Is what I'm feeling a good pain or a bad pain?"

Good pain is that type of sensation we feel when getting a deep tissue massage. It hurts, but it hurts *so good*. We can feel the therapist is releasing trigger points and restricted tissue. Our nervous system is still calm and our body has a "yes" to the experience.

Bad pain within the context of a massage would be when the therapist is pressing so hard you can't breathe and your whole body is contracted to protect against their pressure. You might say to yourself, "It's going to feel good later," but that may not be true. When bruises are left on the body or the entire massage is spent in a state of contraction, that is not good pain.

In a yoga class, good pain may be the discomfort you experience while stretching your hamstrings. It's a lot of sensation, but you are very clear that it's good sensation and your body is grateful you are doing this. Bad pain would be when the teacher pushes you too deeply into a pose and your back suddenly aches or you feel your hamstring tear. This is unfortunately a more common experience than it should be and is often a result of the teacher believing that greater flexibility is the goal of the practice and a sign of improvement.

The simplest way to assess for bad pain is to know that it produces an undesired effect. Sticking your hand in a fire or breaking a bone are everyday examples of this. In the therapy world, trying to mobilize a frozen shoulder (adhesive capsulitis) to a particular range of motion way before it's ready is another example. Yes, eventually we want the shoulder to regain its full range, but if we push it too far too quickly, it will react and tighten up. This can create excessive pain in the moment and even damage the joint further.

To know in your own body if you are feeling good pain or bad pain during stretching or exercise takes intelligence. Intelligence is your ability to listen to the innate wisdom of the body, which requires presence and the cultivation of sensitivity and intuition. Sensitivity allows us to attune to the physical sensations we are feeling as well as the emotions that accompany them. Intuition offers insight into the nature of the experience and its beneficence or maleficence. Ultimately, intelligence means tapping into and trusting your inner knowing.

When working with an injury, it's also important to have knowledge about the biomechanics behind it. This knowledge could come from an educated yoga teacher, physical therapist, chiropractor, or any other movement professional. It's important to ask for support when working with pain—we do not have to go it alone.

Kinesiophobia: Fear of Movement

In 1983, Lethem *et al.* proposed the fear-avoidance model (Figure 2.2).[35] Their goal was to identify why chronic low back pain develops in some patients without pathology while it doesn't in others. They found that fear and avoidance of pain lead to a perpetuation of the original discomfort.

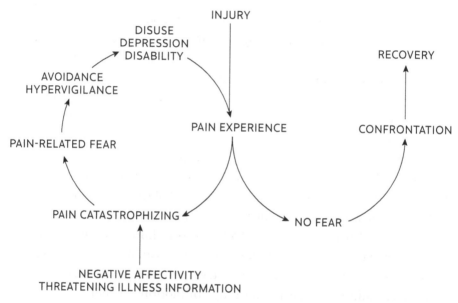

FIGURE 2.2 FEAR-AVOIDANCE MODEL

Vlaeyen and Linton furthered the study in 2000 by proposing when someone is faced with physical pain or injury, they generally have two choices: avoidance or confrontation.[36] Confrontation is a result of not having fear and leads to a significantly quicker recovery. Avoidance puts someone on a path of pain catastrophizing, fear, disuse, disability, depression, and reinjury.

Their term for fear of movement is kinesiophobia. Ishak *et al.* define kinesiophobia as "a state where an individual experiences excessive, irrational, and debilitating fear of physical movement and activity as a result of a feeling of susceptibility to painful injury or reinjury." This fear of movement can inhibit a patient's participation in important rehabilitation activities and may even affect their overall mobility.[37] Thus that fear of movement/pain can be more incapacitating than the experience of pain itself. Preventing a build-up of anxiety that could lead to catastrophizing is yet another reason why empowering ourselves to move immediately after an injury can dramatically impact the healing process. This takes courage and a willingness to face ourselves on both the physical and psychological levels.

Fear of movement is probably the number-one thing I see in people who come to me with acute injuries. When asked if they've done anything to work with their pain yet, the common response is "No. I don't want to make it worse." They are unaware that moving a joint within a pain-free range of motion and including the muscles that have been stressed has been studied and proven to be the most effective treatment in healing. The key, again, is pain-free.

There is, however, a more complex type of pain in the healing process that is not felt in the moment but appears and worsens hours later. This kind of pain can lead to kinesiophobia, which is understandable. It's here that intelligence is especially important. By leaning into and developing a sensitivity to our body's needs, we reduce our potential for this kind of occurrence. If it does happen, we know not to do those exercises the next day and to try something else. This is an act of maturity and responsibility for our own healing.

What is Stretching?

Stretching is an important aspect of the yoga asana practice but is certainly not the only aspect. Yoga incorporates strength techniques, balance acquisition, postural adjustments, breath awareness, and other tools, as well.

The general goals of a stretching routine include improved joint range of motion, decreased muscle tension, improved circulation, relief of pain, prevention of injury, and improved athletic performance. Stretching is commonly used by athletes, dancers, martial artists, gymnasts, and anyone in a rehabilitative process. Physical therapists worldwide incorporate stretching into their clinical treatments for its analgesic affect and ability to increase flexibility.[38]

Stretching focuses on increasing the length of the musculotendinous unit, thus increasing the distance between a muscle's origin and insertion. When we stretch a muscle, we are also affecting other structures such as the joint capsules, fascia, the nervous system, and endocrine system.

Knowledge of the effectiveness of stretching can be determined by increase in joint range of motion. For example, after stretching the hamstring, which is a hip extender, you may notice a greater degree of hip flexion, indicating the hamstring has become looser. Reduction of pain and increased freedom of movement are also indicators.

Very interestingly, however, it is not clear whether the muscles we are stretching are actually increasing their elasticity or we are creating a greater tolerance to the sensations experienced by stretching. Multiple studies of healthy adult individuals ranging from four to six weeks have all concluded that increased range of motion after hamstring stretching was due to stretch tolerance and not to muscle extensibility.[39] All of the studies did show an increase in range of motion, however, thus validating the efficacy of stretching regardless of the scientific reasoning behind it.

Types of Stretching

There are three main types of stretching:

1. static
2. dynamic
3. pre-contraction.

Static stretching is by far the most traditional and what we are used to in yoga. This involves holding a specific position for an extended period of time to a degree where a stretch is felt. All hatha yoga is based on this. More recently, yin yoga has created a relaxing and meditative system where each pose is held for 3–5 minutes. This is congruent with the restorative practices taught by B.K.S. Iyengar, where particular postures are aided by props and held for even longer periods of time.

Static stretching can be done either passively or actively. Passive stretching, as in *supta padangustasana* (reclining hand-to-big-toe pose) (Figure 2.3), involves the use of an external object to aid in the stretch. External objects could be straps, blocks, bolsters, walls, gravity, or even a friend who is holding you in the stretched position.

Active stretching uses muscular contraction to create a stretch. This is done by engaging the motor control system and using something called reciprocal inhibition. Reciprocal inhibition is a law that describes the relaxation of the muscles on one side of the joint to accommodate the participation on the other. If we practiced *supta padangustasana* again, this time without the strap and solely by holding the leg in the air through the strength of our hip flexors, we would be actively stretching the hamstrings and sciatic nerve. Active stretching may not be the best name since the primary focus of a pose like this is the neuromuscular activation of the agonist (the hip flexors in *supta padangustasana*), but it is a form of stretching and very helpful in gaining muscular control.

In the seminars I teach, I often describe it as "muscular activations that aid in relaxation of the antagonist."

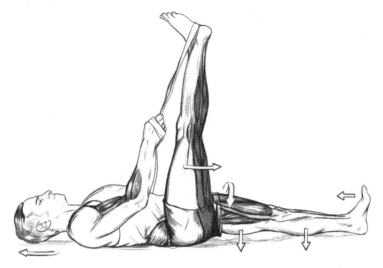

FIGURE 2.3 *SUPTA PADANGUSTASANA* (RECLINING HAND-TO-BIG-TOE POSE) WITH A STRAP

When assessing range of motion as therapists, it is important to understand our client's passive range of motion (PROM) and active range of motion (AROM). A person's PROM shows an ability for their joint to reach a certain range with assistance. Their AROM shows their ability to achieve it on their own through motor control and strength.

Ideally, PROM and AROM should be within 10–15 degrees of each other. When they are not, it shows we are looser than we are strong. Our body has a capacity to reach a certain range, but we don't have the ability to control it. Balancing these two reduces our overall risk of injury.

Dynamic stretching can also be broken down into two categories: active dynamic and ballistic.

Active dynamic stretching involves moving a joint through its full range of motion and repeating it several times. This method has been espoused by the Functional Anatomy Seminars team and their founder, Andreo Spina. They teach that a muscle functions best in its mid-range but that's only because we haven't trained the end ranges. By training the end ranges, we create more articular strength and give our body control over the ranges of motion it has available. We will discuss and practice this in Chapter 5.

Ballistic stretching includes rapid, bouncing movements at the end range of joints. This has been shown to increase injury and will not be discussed further here.

Pre-contraction stretching involves contraction of the muscle being stretched. The most common form of this is proprioceptive neuromuscular facilitation (PNF). PNF was initially created by Dr. Herman Kabat in the 1940s to treat neuromuscular conditions such as polio and multiple sclerosis, but it has now been incorporated into physical therapy, massage, and chiropractic modalities.

There are several types of PNF, including contract relax (CR) and contract-relax agonist contract (CRAC). CR is done by putting the client into a fully stretched position, having them contract isometrically against your pressure between 50–100 percent of their maximum force, and then upon relaxation, pushing them further into the stretch.

CRAC is the same thing except instead of pushing the client into a deeper stretch at the end of their contraction, they engage the antagonist to actively take their joint into a deeper stretch. This requires motor control and is effective if the desired outcome is increasing strength in addition to flexibility.

Two other types of pre-contraction stretching are post-isometric relaxation (PIR), created by neurologist Karel Lewit, and post-facilitation stretching (PFS), created by legendary physical therapist Vladamir Janda.

In PIR, the hypertonic muscle is stretched to the area where resistance is first felt (sub-maximal stretch). A contraction of only 10–20 percent is performed for 5–10 seconds against the therapist's resistance. Upon completion, the therapist stretches the muscle to a new barrier. This is repeated 2–3 times to increase flexibility of the joint.

In PFS, the target muscle is taken to its mid-range level of flexibility and is contracted to its maximum force against resistance. Upon relaxation, the therapist rapidly takes the muscle to its full range for a 15-second stretch.[40] This is repeated 3–5 times. In each repetition, however, the stretched muscle is placed back into its mid-range flexibility instead of its newly found end range. This is different from all the previous techniques, where the muscle is stretched to its maximum range after completion of contraction.

The Stretch Reflex

The stretch reflex is an automatic muscle contraction in response to being stretched. It is designed to be a protective mechanism against muscle strains and tears.

Within the belly of a muscle lies something called a muscle spindle. A muscle spindle is made up of intrafusal fibers and nerve endings encased in connective tissue. These spindles are very sensitive to stretch and cause the muscle to contract when stretched too far or too quickly. The synergistic muscles that produce the same movement are also innervated when the stretch reflex is activated. This strengthens the contraction and allows the muscle to resist with greater capacity.

The stretch reflex also sends an inhibitory signal (via the motor neuron) to the antagonist muscles telling them to relax. Without this, when the stress reflex is triggered and the muscle contracts, the antagonist would then stretch due to reciprocal inhibition. This stretch would cause the stretch reflex to be triggered there as well, causing that muscle to then contract. The result would be both muscles contracting at the same time.

When the contraction from the stretch reflex is emphasized through an isometric, as in CR, it tricks the nervous system into thinking it has control and is safe. This calms down the reflex and allows the muscle to be stretched as much as 15 degrees more than before. In essence, isometrics to a stretched muscle are a way to override the stretch reflex and increase flexibility.

Incredibly, range-of-motion increases have also been seen *bilaterally* with pre-contraction stretching.[41] This points to a possible neurological phenomenon and the interaction between the hemispheres of the brain. As one of my teachers used to say, "If you are having trouble doing an action on one side of the body, let the proficient other side teach it how."

Golgi tendon organs

Golgi tendon organs (GTOs) are proprioceptors that are located in the tendon adjacent to the myotendinous junction. GTOs and muscle spindles work together to regulate muscle stiffness. In contrast to the muscle spindle, however, the GTO causes a muscle to relax when it is stimulated.

GTOs are cool because they are activated when a muscle is contracted *or* stretched. When a muscle is contracted against a force it can't manage, the GTO is triggered and sends a signal to the muscle to relax. This is called autogenic inhibition and prevents the muscle from being injured.

GTOs also become active somewhere around the seven-second mark in a static stretch. When this happens, they send inhibitory signals to the muscle spindle and stretch reflex. This allows the muscle to relax and stretch deeper.

How Long to Stretch For

There is varying research about the effect of duration on stretching. It appears that 30 seconds of hamstring stretching is significantly better than 15, but the difference between stretching for 30 seconds and 60 seconds on hamstring pliability is insignificant.[42] The largest determining factor is not necessarily how long an individual stretch is for but the amount of time spent in a stretch during a given period. Six stretches of 30 seconds (totaling 180 seconds) and four stretches of 45 seconds (also totaling 180 seconds) yield similar results.[43] Note that these are similar results to the effectiveness of isometric loading on tendinopathies.

None of these studies, however, have examined the effect of longer-held poses past one minute. In addition, all of them assessed only a straight leg raise on the sagittal plane after performing *supta padangustasana*, another sagittal plane pose.

To truly get the hamstrings to release and the body to mobilize, performing actions on the frontal and transverse planes is also crucial. A pose like *upavistha konasana* (wide-angled seated pose) (Figure 2.4) is an extremely effective hamstring stretch that can incorporate the sagittal, frontal, and transverse planes depending on which variation you do. It asks for core strength in the upright position and allows access to all three hamstrings muscles in the various forward bending aspects. *Supta padangusthasana II* (reclining hand-to-big-toe pose II) (Figure 2.5) works solely on the frontal plane and aids in stretching the semi-membranosis/tendinosis structures. *Supta padangusthasana III* (reclining hand-to-big-toe pose III) (Figure 2.6) works on the transverse plane, incorporates a spinal twist, and even ads a sciatic nerve glide to the mix. All of these poses, in addition to the array of others in the yogic system, provide the framework for the complex structure of the body to open.

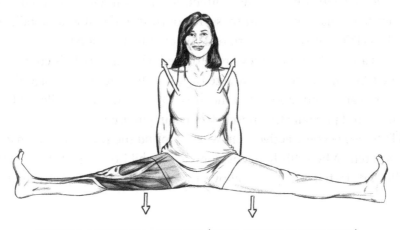

FIGURE 2.4 *UPAVISTHA KONASANA* (WIDE-ANGLED SEATED POSE)

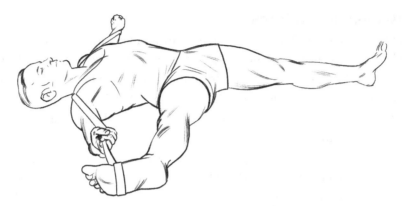

FIGURE 2.5 *SUPTA PADANGUSTHASANA II* (RECLINING HAND-TO-BIG-TOE POSE II) WITH A STRAP

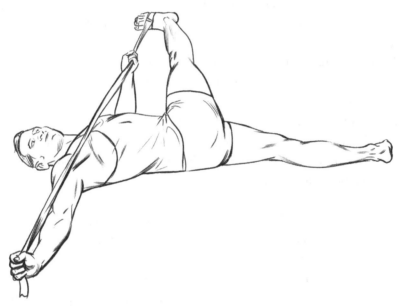

FIGURE 2.6 *SUPTA PADANGUSTHASANA III* (RECLINING HAND-TO-BIG-TOE POSE III) WITH A STRAP

Further studies, I propose, should include poses of anywhere between two and eight minutes and include a skilled yoga teacher to lay out a more thorough and educated plan for increasing mobility.

These studies are also limited in that they only assess the flexibility of the tissues after stretch and nothing else. They are not assessing increases in mindfulness or decreases in anxiety. Due to this, suggesting that there may be no efficacy of stretching for more than 60 seconds is severely limiting and possibly harmful.

Stretching for Athletes

In 2013, *The New York Times* published an article called "Reasons not to stretch."[44] The author, Gretchen Reynolds, references the negative effect that static stretching has on athletic performance if practiced immediately before competition. It is an excellent article backed by extensive research.

In the days that followed, a rash of screams ensued on social media from non-yogis claiming that they were right all these years! Yoga and stretching are bad for you! I was left believing they didn't actually read the article.

As Reynolds references, static stretching prior to exercise has a detrimental effect on muscle strength and performance in runners and jumpers.[45] The term "stretch-induced strength loss" has been coined to indicate this.

There is a lack of understanding as to exactly why this happens, but it has been suggested that a "decrease in muscle stiffness leads to a decrease in the muscle's ability to store and transfer energy."[46] Malachy McHugh, the director of research at the Nicholas Institute of Sports Medicine and Athletic Trauma, says, "There is a neuromuscular inhibitory response to static stretching. The straining muscle becomes less responsive and stays weakened for up to 30 minutes after stretching."[47]

At the end of Reynold's article, which is congruous with another article she wrote in 2008 called "Stretching: The truth,"[48] she states that the research points to dynamic stretching being advantageous before athletic activity. I think this is the paragraph that my friends missed.

Dynamic stretching has consistently been proven to be an effective warm-up compared to static stretching or no stretching at all. Increased sprint speed has been observed in female handball players,[49] as well as total sprint performance in experienced track and field athletes.[50] This increase has been associated with dynamic stretching preparing the athlete for a more optimal switch between concentric and eccentric contraction along with increasing proprioception.

If you have ever gone to a professional baseball game, you'll have seen some of the players doing what is called a "straight leg march" or "toy soldier leg kicks" before the game. This is an active dynamic exercise where the player walks while attempting to kick their opposite hand. This preps their hamstrings and quadriceps for control over both concentric and eccentric contractions while preparing them for more explosive actions during the game.

On another level, stretching feels good, and participants in a different study stated they felt they were "more likely to perform well when stretching was performed as part of the warm-up, irrespective of the type of stretch."[51] This points to the positive psychological and nervous system benefits of stretching.

Stretching, and yoga specifically, have also been touted by Novak Djokovic, quite possibly the greatest tennis player the world has ever seen, as an important factor in his success. He is one of the most flexible players on the tour and attributes his mental toughness and physical health to his yoga practice. You will commonly see him doing a down dog or cobra pose on the court before a match.

The research, then, does support the inclusion of certain warm-up and stretching techniques implemented prior to physical activity in order to reduce the potential of injury.[52] And clearly, stretching and yoga are not lost arts that cause harm to the average person. The important component is which kind of stretching you use, when you use it, and how long for.

MYTH BUST #5

YOGA IS A COMPLETE EXERCISE PROGRAM

When I first began practicing yoga in 1997, there was little to no talk of combining it with strength training. Yoga was meant to be a complete system that exercised your muscles, relaxed your nerves, increased your respiratory capacity, aided in digestion, and nourished your soul. It could fix any injury, heal any wound, and carry you through life with a perennial smile on your face.

Yoga does create a type of strength that is not found in many other modalities. The yogis speak about prana, or life force, as an inner energy that awakens through the practice. When we put our body into unique positions that twist, stretch, and strengthen the muscles, a presence arises that often gives us more capacity to feel like ourselves in the world.

This, however, does not mean it is a complete physical system or the end-all in preventing injury.

According to the American College of Sports Medicine, physical aptitude is comprised of five components:

1. body composition
2. cardiovascular/aerobic fitness
3. muscular strength
4. muscular endurance
5. flexibility.

Body composition is a term used by doctors to refer to the percentage of fat, bone, and muscle in your body. It is used to determine if one is at a healthy weight for their individual body. Yoga can absolutely influence this, both through its activity and potential effects on lifestyle. A significantly overweight person, however, will not lose weight simply by practicing yoga.

Aerobic translates to "with oxygen," and thus **aerobic fitness** is your body's ability to take oxygen from the atmosphere and use it to produce energy for your muscles. Aerobic exercise is commonly referred to as cardio. Examples of cardio include cycling, jogging, and swimming.

Although more intense yoga practices such as Bikram or Ashtanga can influence cardiovascular/aerobic fitness, it still does not often translate into a greater capacity for the above-mentioned exercises. Aerobic training asks us to get our heart rate up, which trains our bodies to move oxygen and blood to the muscles more efficiently.

Strength is defined as the maximum force a muscle or muscle group can generate at a specific velocity. Strength is created through yoga, both physical and mental. But something like hypertrophy, an increase in muscle mass due to exercise, does not occur. As we get older, our muscle mass declines. This is called sarcopenia and it can be as much as 1–2 percent each year after the age of 40. Performing strength or resistance training can combat this, in addition to strengthening our bones and preventing osteoporosis.

Hypertrophy training has been proven to improve cardiorespiratory fitness, fat percentage, lean body mass, lipid profile, and systolic blood pressure.[53] Strong muscles also have a greater ability to complete tasks, which means they require less blood and oxygen to move.[54] This causes less strain on the heart and improves general circulation. There is even evidence that successful completion of a push-up test, where one push-up is completed every three seconds for a total of 60 seconds, reduces the risk of musculoskeletal injury.[55]

Strength training has even been shown to significantly increase flexibility in sedentary women,[56] although it did not affect flexibility in a more athletic, younger group.[57] Strength training combined with flexibility training, however, has been proven to create more optimal results in increased flexibility than simply training flexibility alone.[58]

Muscular endurance is the ability of your muscles to contract repeatedly against a force for an extended period of time. The greater your muscular endurance, the more you are able to repeat a particular exercise. Muscular endurance, like many things, is muscle specific. A professional weightlifter who can do 50 bicep curls of 40 pounds may not be able to swim 30 laps in a pool, because they have not trained that specific capacity.

Muscular endurance will increase through repeated and consistent yoga practice. If you're a yogi, you know that the more classes you've gone to, the more your body adapts to the practice and the easier it gets. At first, you go to class because you know it's good for you, then you go to class because you simply love to be there. Increased muscular endurance has also been linked to a decrease in injury risk.[59]

Flexibility is defined as the ability to bend without breaking. Yoga is by far the most effective path for increasing flexibility. The goals of flexibility training have always been increased joint range of motion, decreased muscle tension, improved circulation, pain relief, and injury prevention. Flexibility has not been proven to decrease potential for injury,[60] however, and should be approached with mindfulness and intelligence.

When we consider these five attributes, it becomes clear that if maintaining a complete and healthy physical structure is your goal, yoga is a great resource but needs to be complemented by strength and aerobic/cardiovascular training. The development of muscle mass and cardiovascular health is important for heart function, reduction of injury, and pain management.

CHAPTER 3

The Breath

Over the last few years, the medical world has started to recognize the relationship of the breath to our physical, mental, and emotional states. Physical therapists, chiropractors, and personal trainers are teaching their clients different ways to breathe in their treatments and training sessions. Practitioners are making links between how their clients are breathing and how they feel in both their bodies and lives. This is a wonderful advancement in the therapy world and crucial for looking at the person holistically. Simply looking at someone as a stack of muscles, bones, and ligaments does not provide the full picture of who they are and what they are experiencing.

There has been one problem, however, in this effort to teach new breathing patterns to people without prior training. There is a lack of understanding by many clinicians about how working with the breath can affect the mind and emotions. Random people are being thrust into breathing practices and told they are doing it wrong without having any prior experience or teaching on how to breathe consciously. Some clinicians have only minimal experience themselves with breathwork yet feel they are an authority on the matter and able to instruct their patients in the practice.

When you manipulate the breath, you effect a change in mood and state of mind. Working with the breath has a different impact on the nervous system than stretching a muscle or lifting weights in the gym. Students must be progressed sequentially through a series of breathing techniques before receiving advanced practices.

In 2016, I attended a highly esteemed movement-based seminar that consisted mainly of personal trainers and physical therapists. There were more than 70 people in the class. At the very end, almost as a side note, the teacher instructed us to take as big a breath as we could and hold it as long as we could. They then asked us to expel as much air as we could and hold the breath out as long as we could. We repeated this three times.

The teacher's intention, which was purely physical, was to create a full contraction and a full relaxation of the diaphragm. The diaphragm is the main muscle of respiration, and since so many of us don't take deep inhalations or exhalations, it doesn't get used anywhere near its maximum capacity. The teacher's intention was good. We all need to learn how to use our diaphragms better. Their method of getting there, however, lacked sensitivity and education. After the class ended, the students were spacey, ungrounded, and light-headed. This is hardly the goal of what we are trying to achieve with our breathwork practice.

This type of breath restraint in yoga is called *kumbhaka* and is one of the more advanced forms of breathwork. Pranayama (breathwork) teachers with years of education under their belts will give a variety of preparatory instructions before imparting this level of practice. Techniques to prepare the lungs, ribcage, diaphragm, and especially the mind must be considered before partaking in strong manipulations of the breath. Teaching advanced methods to someone who has not been practicing breathwork is reckless and can affect their mind and nervous system in a negative way.

History of Pranayama

Pranayama was first documented in India around 2500 years ago. The ancient yogis found that certain ways of breathing elicited specific changes in the mind states they were experiencing. Short, erratic, unconscious breaths had a tendency to induce a state of anxiety, whereas slower, more controlled breathing brought about calmness and relaxation.

The *Hatha Yoga Pradipika*, written around the 15th century by Yogi Swatmarama, listed nine different types of pranayamas, all aimed at giving the sadhaka (practitioner) control over their mind and body. They were:

1. *nadi shodhana*: alternate nostril breathing
2. *surya bhedana*: vitality stimulating breath or sun breath
3. *ujjayi*: psychic or victory breath
4. *sitkari*: hissing breath
5. *sitali*: cooling breath
6. *bhastrika*: bellows breath
7. *brahmari*: humming breath
8. *moorcha*: swooning breath
9. *plavini*: gulping breath.

Of note is that Swatmarama listed *kapalabhati*, probably the most practiced form of pranayama today, alongside alternate nostril breathing, as a shatkarma or internal cleansing technique, and not a pranayama. Since it clearly is a pranayama technique, we can safely say that ten and not nine pranayamas are listed in this text.

Also of note is that a variety of claims are made by Swatmarama about the effects of these pranayamas, including the elimination of worms, remedy of an enlarged stomach or spleen, ability to float, and becoming a *kamadeva* or sex god. Reading these claims, and myriads of others made by hundreds, if not thousands, of Indian yogis, gives rise to an understanding of where many yoga myths originated.

It should also be understood that the medicine available and lifestyle of the Indian culture at this time was nothing compared to what it is today. The yogis were doing what they could based on their intense spiritual practices to share their understanding and knowledge. Many of these pranayamas are rarely practiced anymore, and I will only be discussing a few of them. I will also only teach "basic" breathwork techniques because after practicing every single one listed above for many years, I have found them to be unnecessary and their effects to be volatile.

The Breath and the Nervous System

In his 2015 book *Light on Life*, B.K.S. Iyengar said, "If the breath scatters, the mind wanders. If the mind wanders, the breath scatters. So still the breath to still the mind. Mind is the king."[1] The breath and mind are intimately related and in a continual, interchangeable relationship with one another.

The breath has an innate ability to be a diagnostic tool for how we are feeling in any given moment. It can convey if we're anxious, shut down, calm, stable, happy, or present. Because the breath, mind, and nervous system are so intricately linked, staying connected to the breath allows us to regulate our moment-to-moment experience and create a steady foundation for regulating our moods and emotions.

The breath is the only part of the autonomic nervous system (ANS) that we can control. The ANS is also known as the involuntary nervous system because it acts without our need to think about or control it. It is a component of the peripheral nervous system and contains two distinct divisions: the sympathetic and parasympathetic nervous systems.

Both the sympathetic nervous system (SNS) and the parasympathetic nervous system (PNS) innervate cardiac and smooth muscle as well as various endocrine and exocrine glands. Thus, they have a significant influence on the body's homeostasis. They also typically have opposing effects, so increasing the activity in one decreases the activity in the other.

The SNS stimulates the fight-or-flight response. When it is active, it prepares the body for action by increasing oxygenated blood to the tissues, particularly the working skeletal muscles. The SNS also releases adrenaline while dilating the pupils and bronchioles to allow for more light and air to enter the body. It decreases the actions of the stomach, intestines, and gall bladder to direct the energy normally used there to other areas of the body.

The PNS controls the rest-and-digest response. Its main purpose is to conserve energy and promote relaxation and recovery. It slows the heart rate and increases digestion while constricting the pupils and bronchioles to allow our eyes to be calm and the breath to deepen. The practice of yoga asana and pranayama increases parasympathetic activity.

To elucidate how these two systems work, imagine you're walking down the street, minding your own business, when someone jumps out from behind the corner and yells, "SURPRISE!" You jump and immediately, beyond your control, your heart rate increases, breath quickens, and pupils dilate, and there's a surge of adrenaline. This is the fight-or-flight response and the sympathetic nervous system's reaction to fear as it prepares you to either run or defend yourself.

Compare that to a scenario where you wake up in the morning after a good night's sleep, have a wonderful talk with your spouse, make love, and eat a good breakfast. The breath is slow, the eyes are relaxed, and you'll probably go to the bathroom soon. The parasympathetic nervous system is activated here and your body/mind is in a state of calm.

An overactive sympathetic nervous system has been linked to increased bodily inflammation, cardiovascular and ischemic heart disease, hypertension, kidney malfunction, and depression.[2] It is also quite overactive in people with PTSD and has been associated with an increase in domestic violence and aggression.[3]

Slower breathing techniques calm down the SNS while increasing the activity of the PNS. Heart rate variability (HRV) increases alongside feelings of ease, comfort, and relaxation in people who practice controlled, slower breathing.[4] These are all signs of PNS activity.

Within the PNS is a very influential nerve called the vagus nerve (VN). The VN carries 75 percent of all parasympathetic function and is composed of 80 percent afferent (sensory) and 20 percent efferent (motor) nerves. It is the tenth cranial nerve, exits from the medulla oblongata in the brain, travels inferiorly through the heart and lungs, and terminates in the gastrointestinal tract. Because of its interoceptive (sensory) nature, one of its main roles is to communicate information from the gut to the central nervous system. It is pivotal in recent research of the gut–brain axis (GBA).

The GBA is the connection between the brain, gut, and microbiome. It is the bidirectional link between the central nervous system (CNS) and enteric nervous system (ENS). The ENS contains a web of sensory and motor neurons inside the gastrointestinal system that carry feedback to the brain stem, hypothalamus, and limbic system. These systems, in turn, also carry information from the brain that influences activity in the gut. Ease of communication between these two is important in maintaining adequate mental health.

Although diet is probably the most efficient strategy for maintaining a healthy GBA, the vagus nerve can be modulated through breathwork, and slow, controlled breathing has been shown to have an impact on digestive health. Low vagal tone, a byproduct of high stress and overactive SNS, has been observed in irritable bowel syndrome (IBS) patients and people with functional digestive disorders.

The vagus nerve also impacts the lungs, heart, spleen, liver, and kidneys. Because of its profound impact on our entire system, scientists have created devices that stimulate the vagal nerve. They found that electrical vagal nerve stimulation (VNS) was able to help treat epilepsy and also lead to less depression, a decrease in bodily inflammation, and greater cardiovascular health.[5] This shows even more the importance of affecting our VN and PNS through conscious, intentional breathwork.

Slower, rhythmically paced breathing has been shown to have an impact on various parts of the central nervous system, as well. Through the use of an EEG (electroencephalogram: a device that measures electrical activity in the brain), increased alpha power has been consistently observed.[6] Alpha power promotes mental resourcefulness and aids in the ability to accomplish tasks while remaining easeful and calm. It is reliably found to be associated with positive outcomes such as a reduction in anxiety, depression, anger, and confusion.[7]

In 2011, Yu *et al.* found that just 20 minutes of a type of abdominal breathing used in Zen mediation significantly increased oxygenated hemoglobin in the anterior prefrontal cortex (PFC). They also observed a dramatic increase in whole blood serotonin levels and a reported reduction in negative moods by the participants. This suggests further that breathwork can impact our psychological states through the PFC and 5-HT (serotonin) systems.[8]

The way we habitually breathe is influenced by our emotional states. The interaction between respiration and emotion involves a complex dynamic between the brain stem (homeostasis), the cerebral cortex (intention), and specific aspects of the limbic system (emotional processing). Within the limbic system are two areas of extreme importance: the hypothalamus and amygdala.

The hypothalamus is the part of the brain responsible for transforming perception into cognitive experiences. It is the main link between the endocrine and nervous systems. It helps to regulate the ANS, and since the breath is the only part of the ANS we can control, we can affect our hypothalamus by changing our breathing patterns.

The amygdala is connected to each of the respiratory areas and is known to be the most important area of the brain in managing memory, decision making, and emotional responses such as fear, anxiety, and aggression.

When the breath is fast and erratic, a signal is sent to the amygdala which triggers the fight-or-flight response and sends a distress signal to the hypothalamus. The hypothalamus then sends this SNS response to the rest of the body, causing the release of adrenaline, increased heart rate, dilated pupils, and so on.

Now think for a second how someone who breathes in this way on a regular basis may be perceiving their surroundings. There is a high possibility that they will be overly reactive to situations that may not necessarily demand their defenses. This is the case in people with PTSD, but it happens on much smaller levels as well. Simple overreactions to another person's comments happen all the time. This is one of the reasons that it is commonly suggested you "take a breath" or "take ten breaths" before responding to your spouse, boss, or kid in a stressful situation. The controlling of the breath can calm the amygdala and hypothalamus, thus giving us a wider and more appropriate range of responses than the reactionary one we were about to unload.

Anger often tricks us into thinking it feels good, but rarely does it provide us with the results we are looking for. The Buddha said it is like picking up a burning coal and throwing it at someone. It hurts us way before it hurts the other person. Being able to pause, breathe, and calm the nervous system can greatly increase our quality of life. Consistent breathwork brings the nervous system to a more grounded "default setting"—or the familiar place we fall back to in times of stress. This brings about ease in our lives and connects us to our true selves on a more consistent basis.

Our asana practice should be aimed at increasing our body's innate intelligence. Our breathwork practice is aimed at having a positive impact on our nervous system. As little as five minutes a day can effect a significant change. We often overestimate what we can do in a day and underestimate what we can do in a life. By giving just a little daily attention to our breathing patterns, we can set the tone for calmer and more aligned reactions to internal and external stimuli.

The Diaphragm

The main muscle of respiration is the diaphragm. It is a dome-shaped skeletal muscle that separates the thoracic (chest) and abdominal cavities. Despite a common misconception, the diaphragm flattens on inhalation and expands on exhalation. This is confusing because when you take a deep breath, the ribcage lifts. But this is actually due to the increased pressure in the lungs created by the compression of the diaphragm.

If this is counterintuitive to you, you're not alone. But it is easy to understand through a simple visualization.

Right here, after finishing the next paragraph, place your hands on your ribs and close your eyes. Take five slow breaths.

When you breathe in, visualize the diaphragm flattening. When you exhale, visualize the diaphragm doming.

Go do that. It should take less than one minute.

You feel better, yes? A little calmer?

Studying how our bodies move and breathe creates awareness and grounds us in the present moment.

Since the diaphragm compresses—or activates—on inhalation, it can become weak when we do not regularly take full inhalations, just as any muscle becomes weak without regular exercise. Those who experience a shortness of breath and do not take deep inhalations have diaphragms that lack full functionality and are also more likely to have depression later in their lives.[9]

Similarly, when we do not take full exhalations, the diaphragm never returns to a normal resting position and remains holding a degree of tension. We have already established that the breath is the king of the mind, and now, anatomically, I believe we can say the diaphragm is the king of the breath. What this means is that if we do not allow the diaphragm to relax to its capacity, we are also preventing our minds and nervous systems from relaxing. The two are intimately linked.

The ability to use the diaphragm properly allows the secondary muscles of respiration to relax. These are the scalenes and sternocleidomastoid in the neck, along with the pectoralis minor and upper trapezius in the shoulder. All of these assist in elevating the ribcage during inhalation. When someone is conscious of their diaphragm's proper usage while breathing, these muscles can relax and tension can dissipate.

This does not mean that deep breathing is better than shallow breathing. The key is simply awareness. You will find, however, that more awareness begets more versatility with breathing patterns, and thus an ebb and flow between deep and shallow breaths will naturally occur.

Anatomically, the diaphragm is innervated by the phrenic and vagus nerves. Relaxation of the diaphragm through slow-paced breathing activates the PNS and other important vagal properties. In addition to its respiratory functions, the diaphragm also contributes to correct posture, intraabdominal pressure, and stabilization of the spine. Studies have shown that patients with lower back and sacroiliac joint pain have abnormal diaphragmatic movement during regular breathing and decreased diaphragmatic motion during basic weight-bearing limb activity.[10] The clinical implications of this are quite important and one of the main reasons that Chapter 4, on the lower back, emphasizes the breath.

Amazingly, contraction of the diaphragm upon full inhalation has been shown to decrease one's perception of pain.[11] This is perhaps why so many people hold their breath during painful physical or emotional experiences. It allows them a sense of numbness and withdrawal from situations they may not otherwise have the capacity to be fully present for. Breath holding is also shown in people with depression and chronic physical pain, however, and is hardly an effective approach for carrying yourself through life.

Conscious diaphragmatic breathing, on the other hand, has also been shown to significantly reduce pain symptoms in US veterans with back pain by practicing as little as two minutes a day.[12] This demonstrates breathwork's ability to modulate pain and suggests potential implications in the reduction of opioid and other detrimental pain medication.

The diaphragm should thus clearly be considered when treating anyone who is experiencing pain. It is not just a simple muscle of respiration, but is one with complex musculoskeletal and emotional implications.

Diaphragmatic and Thoracic Breathing

When we discuss breathing, we need to consider two types: diaphragmatic and thoracic. Diaphragmatic breathing involves synchronized motion of the abdomen along with the lower and upper ribcage. This kind of breathing optimizes the natural biomechanical flow of breath in the body and is correlated with a reduced resting heart rate, increased postural control, and numerous other health benefits we've already spoken about.[13]

Thoracic breathing involves breathing predominantly from the chest. This is evidenced by the upper ribcage moving before the lower ribcage. Upper thoracic breathing is associated with hyperventilation, postural instability, and decreased air flow into the lungs.[14] When someone is a thoracic breather, they are relying on their secondary muscles of respiration more than they should. A thoracic breather's ribcage will be stuck in an elevated position and the person will have their "shoulders in their ears." Those who go to massage therapists or chiropractors to release their upper back and neck tension will only receive limited results if the actual problem is a dysfunctional thoracic breathing pattern. The only way to truly change it is to learn proper breathing techniques.

A true breathing pattern disorder can be detected when sub-optimal breathing patterns are combined with musculoskeletal symptoms with no apparent cause. Studies have shown that this, and the subsequent increase in sympathetic nervous system activity, also increases the inflammation in the body. The increase in inflammation causes heightened pain sensations. Medical exams can rarely detect anything wrong. The patient in question will often take a round of ibuprofen to decrease the muscle aches, which may work temporarily, but until the root issue is resolved, the problem keeps returning.

This is also similar to the symptoms of a psychosomatic disorder. A psychosomatic disorder, as we described earlier, is a condition where mental and emotional stresses adversely affect the physiological function of the body. Doctors are unable to diagnose any medical condition, and the person is left with excessive thoughts and concerns about what may be going on. In these situations, being able to find an educated breathwork facilitator can make the difference between cycling through various medications or actually accessing the root cause of the issue.

There are two main, *non-pathological* reasons why someone might have a breathing pattern disorder:

- lack of education on proper breathing technique
- mental and emotional difficulties.

Very few people in the world are taught how to breathe properly at a young age. Thankfully, this is beginning to change. The era of yogis that the 1980s and 1990s ushered in has created more conscious parents who are able to instruct their children on mindfulness, breathing, and embodiment. This is certainly something to be applauded.

We have spoken extensively about emotional/mental difficulties and their effect on the breath. Emotional states alter breathing and breathing can alter emotional states. This is a two-way street where both have influence on the other.

Breathing and Athletic Performance

More athletes are understanding the importance of the effect of respiration on performance. This was exemplified by former professional tennis player Andy Roddick around 2012: you could hear him audibly exhale during every shot he hit. He was using his breath to focus his mind and give him more strength and accuracy. Sadly, he still couldn't beat Federer, so I guess the proper breathing fundamentals doesn't override superior athletic capability.

In 2014, Helen Bradley and Joseph Esformes performed a study to assess the effects of the breath on the Functional Movement Screen, or FMS. The FMS, created by Gray Cook, is a set of graded movements used to assess if someone is more or less likely to get injured. Of people studied in this group, the mean score on the FMS was 14.7. Those who scored less than 14.7 were more likely to get injured and those that scored higher than 14.7 were less likely. Of those who scored less than 14.7, 75 percent were classified as thoracic breathers, and 66.6 percent of those who scored greater than 14.7 were classified as diaphragmatic breathers.[15] Thus this study demonstrates that thoracic breathers are more likely to get injured, and illustrates the importance of diaphragmatic breathing on functional movement and injury potential.

In another study, competitive swimmers between the ages of 13 and 20 practiced 30 minutes of breathwork every day for five days per week. They all subsequently exhibited increased respiratory muscle endurance and were able to complete more strokes per breath. This was in addition to a decrease in overall feelings of anxiety (pre-race jitters).[16]

Breathing is the number-one movement pattern we have. It's the first thing we do when we're born and the last thing we'll do before we die. The yogis said that because of this, the breath is something we should study to a great extent. We are now seeing its far-reaching effects on every aspect of our lives.

Nasal Breathing vs. Mouth Breathing

The yogis have long known the positive effects of nasal breathing on our psychospiritual and physical bodies. The pranayamas they taught were all inhaling through the nose and exhaling out of the nose except for two where they inhaled through the mouth and out of the nose. It's quite possible these were created due to the high temperatures in India and the fact that breathing through the mouth cools the air while breathing through the nose warms it. This is evidenced by the transition to mouth breathing that normally occurs when someone is in a sauna for an extended period of time. The body's natural response is to breathe through the mouth to cool the air that's entering the body.

Breathing through the nose warms and humidifies the air we breathe. The hairs within the nose filter out dust, pollen, and other allergens, preventing them from entering the lungs. Because the nose and sinuses are part of the body's immune system, nasal breathing improves our capacity to fight off various respiratory infections. The nose also releases nitric oxide during nasal breathing, which helps to widen the blood vessels and improve oxygen circulation throughout the body.

Mouth breathing can have a variety of deleterious effects on the body. It is considered an abnormal and inefficient adaptation of the breathing mechanism and induces functional, postural, and biomechanical imbalances.[17] It is linked with numerous pathologies including upper respiratory tract infections, asthma, and sleep apnea. In children who mouth breathe, malocclusion—a misalignment of the teeth—occurs and can even affect the way their face develops.[18]

In his book *Breath: The New Science of a Lost Art*, James Nestor documents his experience of undergoing a study at Stanford University to understand the differences between nasal and mouth breathing.

For ten days, Nestor and a colleague had their noses plugged and were only allowed to mouth breathe. Each day they would go through various tests to understand the effects this was having. After only the first night, Nestor's snoring increased by 1300 percent. He had four sleep apnea moments, his blood pressure went up by 13 points, HRV plummeted, and body temperature decreased. By the end of ten days, his snoring had increased by 4800 percent, he was having 25 sleep apnea events per night, his mental clarity was at an all-time low, and his oxygen levels had decreased to 85 percent (95%–100% is normal). When this happens, the blood can't carry enough oxygen to support the body's tissues, and heart failure, physical pain, and depression can occur.

By the time this part of the study concluded, his nasal cavity was so clogged it had to be manually cleaned. After just 24 hours of doing the opposite—taping his mouth and nasal breathing—his blood pressure decreased by 18 points and HRV increased by 150 percent. He had no events of sleep apnea and went from four hours of snoring a night to ten minutes. His mental clarity and overall sense of well-being greatly increased.[19]

The military are also trained in specific types of nasal breathing to reduce stress and increase mental sharpness in dangerous situations. This allows them to keep their heart rate down and manage any fear that may arise. When most of us are huffing and puffing out of our mouths while running up a hill, these trained forces are still maintaining an equal inhalation and exhalation through the nose. The type of breathing they use is called tactical breathing, or box breathing, and will be described later in this chapter.

The Tarahumara tribe in Mexico, probably the world's most elite ultra-marathon runners (brilliantly depicted in Christopher McDougall's book *Born to Run*[20]), are trained from youth to only breathe through their noses by having a few pebbles or a bit of water placed in their mouths while running. This forces them to breathe in and out of the nose even at extreme levels of fatigue. The ability to maintain nasal breathing through such intense physical exertion allows for greater diaphragmatic capacity, less accessory muscle activation, and more athletic endurance.[21]

It will come as no surprise, then, that all the pranayamas taught in this book will be in through the nose and out of the nose. It is not wrong to breathe out of the mouth when you have to. I am not trying to make that taboo. In times of high stress, mouth breathing, or perhaps in through the nose and out of the mouth, can be very helpful. But for diaphragmatic function, nervous system education, quality of life, and yogic training purposes, nasal breathing is a far more effective approach.

Guidelines for Working with the Breath

There are a few important rules to follow when engaging in breathwork practice. The first, outside of nasal breathing, is to never strain or force. The breath should be natural. When more advanced pranayamas are introduced, it is tempting to fit ourselves into what we believe the breath should look and feel like. This often leads to tension, both mental and physical. The key is listening and surrendering.

Should you ever be practicing breathwork and find yourself in a state of physical or psychological tension, return to normal, uncontrolled breathing. Become aware of the state you're experiencing and the breath as it is. Watch only where it travels naturally. Let your nervous system calm down and return to homeostasis.

The Marvel movie *Doctor Strange* has a great quote that exemplifies the path of breathwork. Stephen Strange, a spiritual neophyte trying to find a magical cure for his injured fingers, demands his guru gives him the teachings immediately. His guru, known as the ancient one, observes his impatience and responds by saying, "You cannot beat a river into submission. You have to surrender to its current and use its power as your own."[22] This signifies the direction of our spiritual path and the necessity of preparatory work before advanced technique.

With breathwork, your job is to listen to your nervous system and use the breath the way it is asking. This is a subtle practice and demands a constant alignment between your will and nervous system. When will overpowers the nervous system's needs, anxiety arises. When will and nervous system are harmonized, tranquility and mental alertness awakens. The practitioner is now using the breath's life force as their own.

Where in the Body to Breathe?

Where we breathe may very well be as important as how we breathe. Learning to direct the breath to different regions of the body creates a sense of calmness in the mind and an intimacy with the pathways of the breath. It is as much a type of pranayama as any of the traditional practices.

Although functional diaphragmatic breathing synchronizes motion of the lower abdomen to the lower and upper ribs, that doesn't mean this is the only correct way to breathe. Teaching yourself first to breathe individually into each of these regions is valuable in terms of rib and lung expansion, oxygen intake, and diaphragm control. It also generates concentration and precision of mind.

With your breathwork practice, you can breathe singularly into the lower abdomen, navel, lower ribs, side ribs, sternum (breast bone), and upper ribs. Even when more advanced diaphragmatic breathing practices are introduced, it's important to return to these basic breathing patterns in the same way a master still practices their fundamentals.

The Breathwork Practice: Learning to Breathe into the Body

Breath awareness can happen any moment we are awake. Traditional practice is done in one of the four seats, however: sitting, standing, lying down, or walking. My hope is that the more you practice in these formal positions, the more you bring that to your everyday life. Whether you are in the car, online at the checkout counter, or sitting at your desk using the computer, the opportunity exists to become conscious and aware of how you are breathing.

For formal practice, there are several positions I personally prefer and offer to my students as they begin their journey. These are listed in order of accessibility to the beginner but should still be practiced even by advanced practitioners.

1. Prone *savasana* (corpse pose): 5 minutes

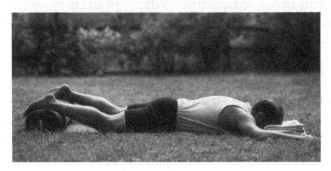

FIGURE 3.1

Lie face down with your forehead supported by a blanket. You will need enough lift to prevent your nose from pressing into the floor but not enough to compress the back of your neck. It is best to have the head straight, but if you can't find comfort, you may turn the head. The bolster under the ankles takes pressure off the lower back.

Begin by breathing into your belly and feeling the pressure of it against the floor. This will be natural. Allow your head to rest. After one minute, start breathing into your lower side ribs. You will feel them expand outwardly as well as up towards your head and perhaps also into the floor. Focus on this for 1–2 minutes. See if you can then feel the sensation of your lower and upper back moving while breathing. Do not force anything or make yourself tense. If you fall asleep or totally space out into some restful daze, let it be. Your body needed it. If you stay present and attentive, that is great as well.

2. Supported *savasana* (corpse pose): 5–8 minutes

A. LIE FLAT ON THE GROUND WITH A BLANKET
UNDER YOUR HEAD (FIGURE 3.2)

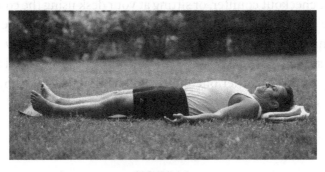

FIGURE 3.2

B. LIE OVER A SUPPORTED PRANAYAMA SET-UP (FIGURE 3.3A, B, C)

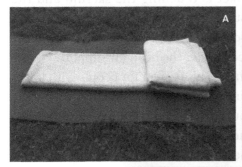
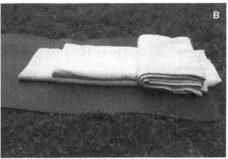
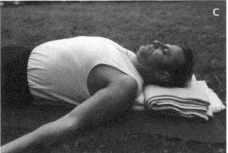

FIGURE 3.3A, B, C

C. CALVES ON THE CHAIR: ESPECIALLY GOOD FOR PEOPLE WHO HAVE LOWER BACK PAIN AS THIS TAKES PRESSURE OFF THE DISCS (FIGURE 3.4)

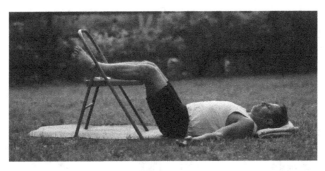

FIGURE 3.4

There are four supported *savasana* set-ups that I like the most. The first is a simple *savasana* with a blanket under the head (Figure 3.2). The second is with a rectangularly folded blanket to support the spine and head (Figure 3.3a). The bottom edge of the blanket is placed at the level of the kidneys, near the thoracolumbar junction, to provide support. Then one blanket is placed under the head.

The third supported *savasana* is the one I use the most. This is a stacked blanket set-up where the lower blanket is touching the sacrum and the top blanket is placed so it rests against the kidneys/thoracolumbar junction (Figure 3.3b, c). This set-up gives a little lift to the chest and allows for easier lung expansion. There is a blanket placed under the head for support.

The fourth is with the calves on a chair. This is great for people with lower back pain as it alleviates compression in the spine (Figure 3.4).

Being by placing your hands on your belly and allow yourself to breathe into your hands (Figure 3.5a, b). Feel the sensation of the abdomen rising and falling. Do this for 1–2 minutes. Become acquainted with the feeling of gentle, slow, belly breathing.

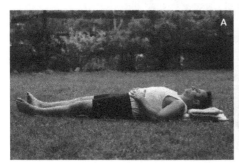
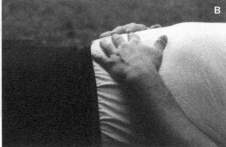

FIGURE 3.5A, B

Then move the hands up to the lower ribs (Figure 3.6a, b). Your palms should be touching the sides of your ribs and the fingers pointing towards each other but not touching. Breathe three times into your fingertips. This is just to familiarize yourself with the ability to direct the breath where you want to.

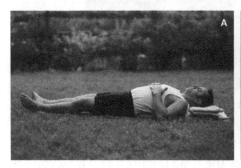
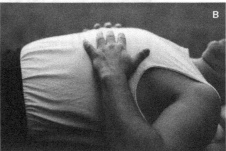

FIGURE 3.6A, B

Now bring your hands a little wider onto the ribs (Figure 3.7). Breathe into your palms. This gives you a kinesthetic experience of expanding your ribs laterally, as opposed to anteriorly and superiorly (forward and upwards) as we normally do. Do this for 2–3 minutes. This is important for ribcage expansion, diaphragm function, intercostal space, mental clarity, and lower back pain. It's this type of breathing that is considered "correct" by many new-age practitioners. It's essential to understand its value but not to lock ourselves into some narrow thinking that this is the only way to breathe.

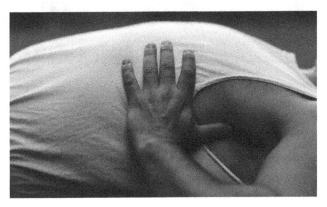

FIGURE 3.7

Bring your hands now as high as you can on your side ribs (Figure 3.8a). You can even invert them if that's easier for you (Figure 3.8b, c). Breathe into this uppermost part of your ribs, near the armpit. Do this three times.

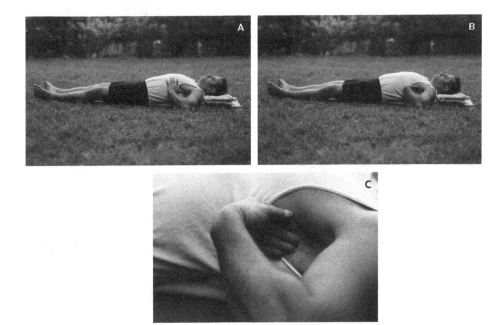

FIGURE 3.8A, B, C

Now take your arms out to your sides (Figure 3.9). This lifts your ribs and allows for even greater access into the upper intercostal region. Breathe here three times.

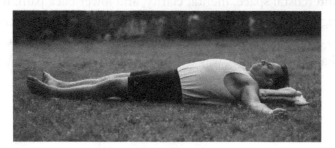

FIGURE 3.9

This completes one supine breathwork cycle. To see this cycle with the calves on a chair, see Figures 3.10a–f. At any time, you may repeat this whole cycle, or if you feel like only breathing into one of these areas, that's also great practice. The key, as always, is to listen to your nervous system and not override its needs with your desires.

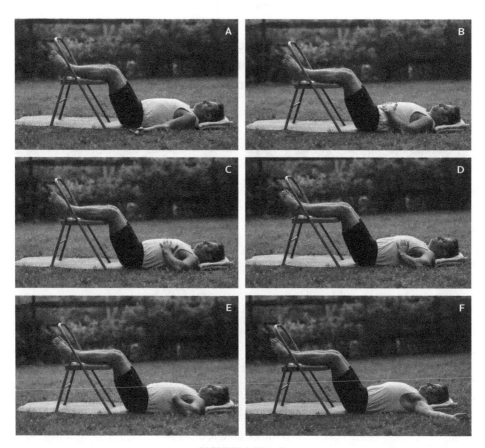

FIGURES 3.10A–F

3. Seated
A. CROSS-LEGGED ON A CUSHION (FIGURE 3.11)

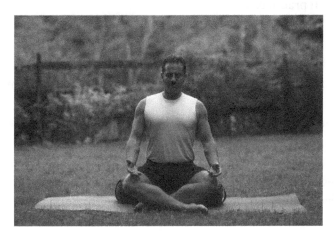

FIGURE 3.11

B. UPRIGHT ON A CHAIR (FIGURE 3.12)

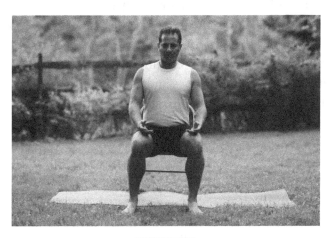

FIGURE 3.12

As you get more comfortable, you may progress to practicing while sitting, either cross-legged on a cushion or upright in a chair. Set a timer for five minutes and see if you can watch your breath for that period. Watch the rising and falling of the belly and/or the ribs.

Another point of attention could be the flow of air through your nostrils. This would be more akin to traditional meditation than a controlled form of pranayama. When you breathe in, the air enters through the lower portion of your nostrils, and when you breathe out, it leaves through the upper portion. Most people are not aware of this, but if you practice for just ten seconds right now, you'll see. The breath is also cooler when it enters your nose than when it leaves. Observing just this flow for five minutes is a very powerful concentration practice.

A Tip on Meditation from the Buddha

In one of the Buddha's most important and possibly simplest teachings, he says:

> When the yogi breathes in, he knows he is breathing in. When he breathes out, he knows he is breathing out. When he breathes in deeply, he knows he is breathing in deeply. When he breathes out deeply, he knows he is breathing out deeply. When he breathes in shallowly, he knows he is breathing in shallowly. When he breathes out shallowly, he knows he is breathing out shallowly.

At no point does the Buddha tell us to breathe in a certain way or that the lower ribs must expand laterally or we're doing it wrong. He is only saying that the honest practitioner knows what is happening and when.

The next time you want to meditate, try this: Take five minutes, sit down, and observe your breath. Whether it is shallow, deep, fast, or slow, say to yourself upon inhalation, "I am breathing in..." and upon exhalation say, "I am breathing out..." See how it goes and how you feel after. Remember, the mind will always wander. Getting it to stop is not the goal. The goal is simply awareness.

Types of Pranayamas

1. Three-part breath

The three-part breath is probably the oldest form of breathwork we know. It is a simple breath that teaches you to follow the natural path the breath should flow in the body. Begin by breathing into the abdomen and allowing it to expand. When the belly gets full of air, breathe upwards into your lower ribs and then your chest. Do not lift your shoulders as this engages the accessory muscles of respiration too much. Exhale. This completes one cycle. Repeating this 3–4 times or for 3–4 minutes will aid in overall relaxation.

2. Box breathing

Box breathing is a technique where the practitioner breathes in for four seconds, holds for four seconds, breathes out for four seconds, and holds out for four seconds. Traditionally, this is accompanied by visualizing the creation of box with each segment of the breath. As you breathe in, visualize a line going vertically; as you hold the breath the line goes horizontally, and so on until you've completed one full cycle and created a box. The visualization helps with concentration but is not necessary for the practice.

Box breathing and tactical breathing are both used by the military. Tactical breathing is a conscious slowing down of the breath without the use of a breath hold. It is used in acute high-pressure situations to reduce stress and maintain psychomotor and cognitive performance. "Box breathing," says Mark Divine, a former Navy SEAL, "is more of a daily practice used for stress management, emotional awareness and mental sharpness. It was instrumental in saving my life several times in crises. I was able to remain calm and focus clearly to avoid reactionary thinking or panic."[23]

3. Cardiac coherent breathing

Cardiac coherent breathing is a type of breathwork where the inhalation and exhalation are 5.5 seconds each. This has an even greater effect on heart rate variability than other slow breathing techniques.[24] The average person breathes 12–14 times per minute, but in cardiac coherent breathing, that is reduced to around five. This allows for more lung expansion, diaphragmatic control, and vagally mediated nervous system responses.

4. *Nadi shodhana* (alternate nostril breathing)

There are many ways to practice *nadi shodhana*. All of them assume the hand position shown in Figure 3.13a) while closing one nostril at a time. The right nostril will be closed with the right thumb and the left nostril is closed with the ring and pinky fingers. *Nadi shodhana* is best practiced while seated so either the position shown, raised on a bolster, or on a chair will be best. Your opposite hand is placed on the thigh, either palm face up or down (Figure 3.13b, c).

TECHNIQUE 1

Sit up straight and close the left nostril with the ring and pinky finger while the right thumb gently rests on the right nostril. Take a full inhalation and exhalation through the right nostril. Repeat 3–5 times or to your level of comfort. Now close the right nostril with the right thumb while the ring and pinky finger rest on the left nostril. Take 3–5 full inhalations and exhalations. This is a preparatory step for *nadi shodhana*.

TECHNIQUE 2

Sit up straight and close the left nostril with the ring and pinky finger while the right thumb gently rests on the right nostril. Take a full inhalation through the right nostril, then close it with the right thumb. Exhale fully through the left nostril. Inhale fully through the left nostril and close it with the ring and pinky fingers. Exhale fully through the right nostril. This completes one cycle. Repeat 1–5 times.

TECHNIQUE 3

Combine box breathing and alternate nostril breathing. Breathe through the right nostril for a count of four. Close both nostrils and hold the breath for four seconds. Exhale through the left nostril for four seconds and hold the breath out for four seconds. Breathe in through the left nostril for four seconds. Close both nostrils for four seconds. Breathe out through the right nostril for four seconds. This completes one cycle. Repeat 1–3 times.

It has been my experience that the mind clears best with technique 3 and that no more than three repetitions are needed. Remember that the key to success is to listen to your nervous system and to never strain or force. There are times that I practice and one repetition is more than enough; other times, I like a set of three. Attuning yourself to your individual needs becomes a developed skill of self-introspection.

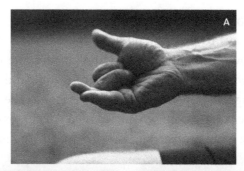

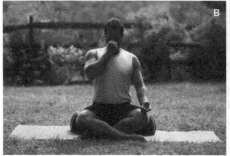
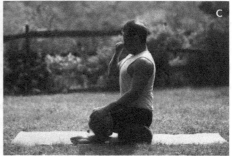

FIGURE 3.13A, B, C

Note: There are more variations of timing for the inhalation, exhalation, and breath holds in *nadi shodhana*. Some books espouse a 4–7–8 breath, meaning to breathe in for four seconds, hold for seven, and exhale for eight. Some even say 4–16–8. All of these can be explored, but my experience is that the techniques described above are the safest and most effective.

Which Pranayama to Practice?

As always, the best breath for you is the one that calms your nervous system and awakens your mind. At times, simple three-part breathing may be exactly what you need. At others, the focus created by box breathing or *nadi shodhana* may be perfect. Some days, cardiac coherent breathing at 5–6 seconds per inhalation-exhalation without any pause may calm your sympathetic nervous system and activate your parasympathetic. And other days, 5–6-second breaths may be too much or even too little. The key to success, as I've said since the beginning of this chapter, is to listen and surrender to your nervous system's needs.

When to Practice

Although it's nice to have a formal breathwork practice every morning or evening, this is not the only way to go about it. Some people love to practice first thing in the morning as a way to set their mood for the day. Others love to practice before bed and find that it helps them sleep longer and more deeply. Both of these are great.

Another method is to disperse short breathing sessions throughout your day. With the stresses of life and all its demands, we often forget to breathe. Doing 1–3 sets of box breathing, belly breathing, cardiac coherent breathing, simple mindfulness of breath, or whatever you'd like can be influential in how you feel throughout your day and how you respond to different situations. The key to this is finding a rhythm that works for you.

A Note on One Other Form of Breathwork: Holotropic Breathwork

Holotropic breathwork was created by Stanislav Groff in the mid-1970s. Groff had been a psychedelic researcher at the Psychiatric Research Institute in Prague where he facilitated experiences for participants with LSD, psilocybin, and mescaline. Over many years, he observed great transformations in his patients but also found that some would experience deeply unpleasant feelings while coming down. He began guiding them deeper into the "darkness" they were feeling and found that some spontaneously began breathing much faster and were going through various cathartic experiences. These ranged from shaking, coughing, screaming, and crying to actually vomiting. At the end of these releases, they felt calm, centered, and clear.

Groff and his wife Christina decided to create a system of breathwork to help facilitate deep psychological transformation without the use of psychedelics. Holotropic breathwork (HB) involves voluntary hyperventilation through rapid, prolonged, mindful, and deep over-breathing that brings the practitioner into a non-ordinary state of mind. Practitioners commonly experience cathartic events similar to what Groff observed in his patients on LSD.

Holotropic breathwork is often done in large groups where there are "Breathers" and "Sitters." The Breathers are those doing the practice while the sitters are there to hold space and provide undivided attention and support to their partner. This can also be done in a one-on-one psychotherapeutic setting.

HB has been shown to significantly reduce avoidance behaviors and allow practitioners deeper access to their emotions.[25] This is likely because HB is a somatic experience and doesn't involve psychological processing of previous traumas. It is much easier to access the body than to penetrate the walls in the mind. HB has thus been shown to create higher self-awareness and self-transcendence. This increase in self-transcendence allows the breather to become more patient and equanimous in the face of conflict and struggle.[26] It is quite possible that people who have not responded well to traditional psychotherapy could respond well to HB.[27]

Holotropic breathwork will obviously not be taught in this book, but if you feel inclined to learn about it, I encourage you to do so.

Breathwork and Asana Practice

One of the most concrete ways to connect to your breath is through the movements in the yoga practice. Forward bends open the back portion of your body to receive the breath, and back bends open the front. Twists teach you to stay calm with less ability to take in air. This means that you can use individual postures to teach your breath to move to areas that are difficult to reach in the classical meditation positions.

Here is one sequence you can try, along with the corresponding areas that become accessible for the breath in each position. Breathe consciously in each pose. Don't worry about creating perfect physical alignment. Your focus will be on the breath and maintaining comfort in your body. You can stay in each pose for as long as you like. This practice, in general, can completely change your mood and breathing pattern for the day.

Child's pose

Child's pose gives you direct access to your upper back and chest. Watch the breath move here. After a small amount of time, you should also be able to direct the breath into the side ribs and abdomen.

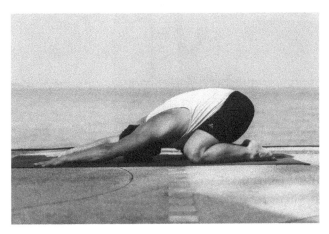

FIGURE 3.14

Down dog

Down dog allows you to take longer breaths into your belly. Since the abdomen is elongated, the breath can be very calming for the organs. The chest is also easily accessed in this position as well, but don't feel that you have to force it. Elongated abdominal breathing is very powerful.

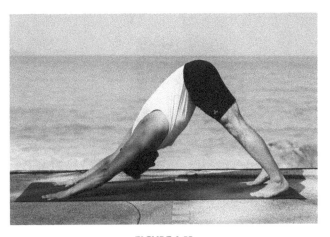

FIGURE 3.15

Uttanasana (standing forward fold)

Watch the breath move from your abdomen to your upper back and chest.

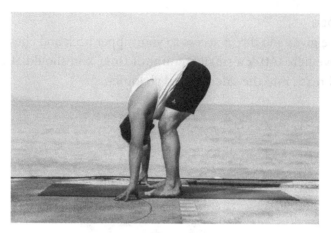

FIGURE 3.16

Tadasana (mountain pose)

The abdomen will normally grip upon exhalation to ensure that we are expelling enough air. Do that—slowly—several times, as we do for plank pose in Chapter 4. Then see if you can resist that and keep the abdomen soft upon exhalation. Your breath will be shallower at first. Use this to still your mind and calm your nerves.

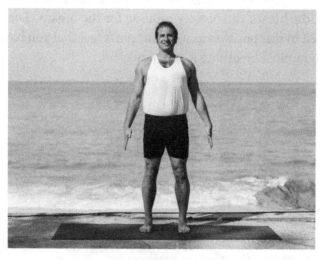

FIGURE 3.17

Virabhadrasana II (warrior II)

This pose allows you to breathe into the upper side ribs and chest. The main reason for this is so that the arms are lifted. If you took *tadasana* with your arms outreached as they are in *virabhadrasana II*, you should have the same results.

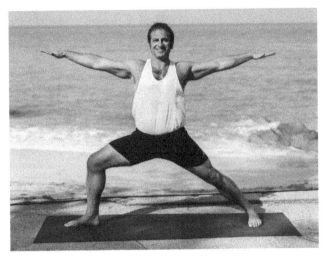

FIGURE 3.18

Prasarita padottanasana (wide-legged forward fold)

Place your hands on the floor in front of you. This pose gives you direct access to your side ribs and upper back. Breathe into these areas, expanding them as much as you can.

Prasarita padottanasana allows you to direct the breath where you'd like to. You can breathe only into the belly or you can take a smooth three-part breath into the abdomen and then upwards into the chest. Play with it and feel into what works best for you in a given moment.

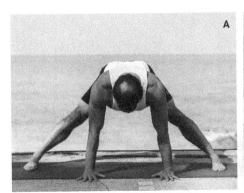 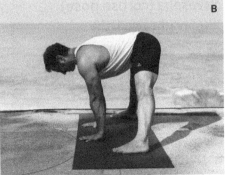

FIGURE 3.19A, B

Supta dandasana (reclined staff pose)

Sit in *dandasana* with your legs in front of you. Lean backwards and place the elbows on the ground. Lift the chest and tilt the head backwards to your level of comfort. Breathe into your chest, expanding your ribs.

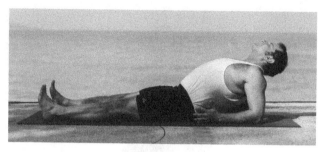

FIGURE 3.20

Upavistha konasana (wide-angled seated pose)

Take a complete three-part breath, breathing first into the belly and tracking it upwards into the ribs.

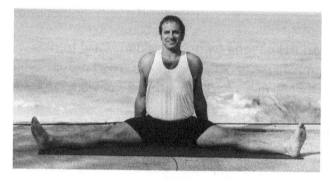

FIGURE 3.21

Savasana (corpse pose)

Just breathe regularly.

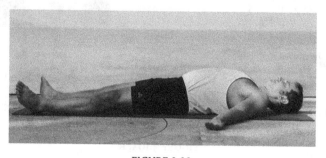

FIGURE 3.22

PART II

APPLYING THE TEACHINGS

The Movement Practices

The following practices are designed to help you build strength and mobility throughout your entire body. They have been created after years of trial and error with me and thousands of students. As with everything in this book, the key to success is intelligence. It is up to you to listen to your body and fine-tune each pose to make it yours. Specific directions are given as guidelines, but minor adaptations are often necessary to find the exact nook or cranny of your body that needs attention. Always feel free to adjust.

Practicing once and hoping for a miracle is not the way to heal from an injury. These techniques take repetition, and it is recommended to do whatever practice you are doing 3–4 days a week. You absolutely may do more, but it's important to set realistic goals for yourself. Some people can practice every day without fail, and others will only be able to commit to a Monday–Wednesday–Friday schedule. Both are fine and will yield results.

In Patanjali's *Yoga Sutras*, he speaks about *tapas*. Tapas is the third niyama, or spiritual discipline, and translates to internal fire. This is the fire that arises in anyone with passion and dedication. It's something that develops naturally and is also something for us to cultivate. In order to heal an injury, we must apply tapas/discipline to a specific practice. This takes time, patience, and repetition.

Tapas arises when one feels *inspiration.* Inspiration with movement therapy comes when a pose or an action is performed and immediate results are felt. Any combination of an increase in strength or flexibility or a decrease in pain will inspire someone to continue doing that same exercise later. The number of times I've seen clients who have been in physical therapy for months but eventually left because they were repeatedly given the same cookie-cutter exercise without seeing any benefit is higher than I'd like to admit. It takes finesse and knowledge to be able to prescribe and adjust movement as medicine. Communication with your student and sensitivity to their needs, successes, and failures are critical in the therapeutic process.

It is also important to empower our students to take responsibility for their healing. When people are fully reliant on us to heal them, there is a power dynamic that rarely results in therapeutic success. Giving them the tools and understanding to do the work themselves (under our guidance) encourages self-agency. To do this, we must be proficient in what we're sharing and have knowledge of what we're treating. That comes with practice, education, and trial and error.

Understanding what muscles are moving in your body and where you should be feeling something activate gives you confidence and an important form of embodiment. It never ceases to amaze me how many people don't know where their diaphragm is or which muscle is the hamstring and which one is the quadricep. This body we live in should be explored and understood.

CHAPTER 4

Anatomy of the Lower Back

Problems of the low back are the number-one musculoskeletal complaint that brings people to doctors. It is estimated that around 80 percent of Americans will at some point complain of back pain in their lives.[1]

In studies conducted by the Institute for Health Metrics and Evaluation (IHME), lower back pain was *globally* the leading cause of disability in both 1990 and 2017.[2] According to data from the National Institute of Health (NIH), back pain costs the US between $560 billion and $635 billion annually. And the American Chiropractic Association (ACA) states that if you include lost wages, American citizens spends over $100 billion yearly on back pain alone.[3]

The numbers are staggering.

When the low back gets injured, the common understanding is that we must "strengthen our core." For many, this means the abdominal muscles, which include the rectus and transversus abdominus, and internal and external obliques. While strengthening these muscles can certainly be beneficial, thinking of this as "the core" is an outdated view and one that needs redefining.

We all would love to develop a six pack, but doing so will do little to substantively affect your lower back pain. Strengthening these muscles relieves pressure on the lower back, but solely focusing on the abs will also inhibit the low back from being able to strengthen. This is because of reciprocal inhibition, a dynamic where the contraction of one side of a muscle group creates the relaxation of the opposite side.

In all my years as a therapist, I have never seen someone freed of their low back's distress solely from an increase in abdominal strength.

Low back pain has become more prevalent in the last 50 years. With the advent of people spending their entire day sitting at a desk or commuting long hours in a car, the spine is forced into a flexed position for extended periods of time. This weakens the lower back muscles and they lose their capacity for support and stability.

One of my students, a Pilates teacher in New Zealand, had experienced low back pain for years. She spent hours on end strengthening her abs to no avail. When she finally went to an orthopedist and got an MRI, he told her that her multifidi—the very small spinal stabilizing muscles that run up and down the entire spine—were "wasted."

Studies show that people with chronic low back pain often have multifidus atrophy coupled with fatty replacement.[4] Put simply, the muscles literally become fat due to lack of use.

The multifidi are unique muscles in that they are able to produce a large amount of force over a small area. This makes them ideal for stability as opposed to movement, and thus they are key factors in healing lower back pain.

For this reason, targeting the posterior chain—the muscles lining the back of your body—is crucial for working with any kind of low back injury. As Eric Goodman and Peter Park say in their fantastic book *Foundation*, "For every exercise you do for the front of your body, you should do at least four for the back."[5]

Strengthening the posterior chain involves not only the multifidus but also the glutes, hamstrings, and erector spinae. Especially for yoga practitioners who spend so much time stretching their hamstrings, twisting, and rotating their backs, this is often a counterintuitive approach that yields great results and a lot of good, sore muscles.

There are three gluteal muscles: gluteus maximus, gluteus medius, and gluteus minimus. These three muscles work in synergy to keep us upright and bipedal as opposed to quadrupedal like most other mammals.

The gluteus maximus (GM) is one of the largest and strongest muscles in the body. Along with keeping us upright, its main job is extension of the hip. The GM tends towards inhibition and weakness, and thus the term 'gluteal amnesia' has become quite prevalent. This is mostly due to the amount of time we spend sitting in cars and at desks instead of spending our days outside farming, hunting, and partaking in many of the outdoor activities our ancestors enjoyed.

Weakness in the GM is associated with sacroiliac joint and lumbopelvic pain.[6] When the GM doesn't fire properly and take the hip into extension, other muscles such as the hamstrings and erector spinae, also hip and spinal extenders, must contract in compensation. This is called synergistic dominance, and the imbalance between these muscles can lead to hamstring tears and back ache.[7]

Dysfunction in the GM also contributes to knee pain since the iliotibial band (ITB), which inserts onto the lateral portion of the tibia, is just the fascial continuation of the gluteus maximus, gluteus medius, and tensor fascia latae.[8]

ANATOMY OF THE LOWER BACK   **103**

When any of these three muscles are weak, it can put extra pressure on the ITB and pull on the knee.

I have always valued the importance of a strong gluteus maximus in relation to low back health, so much so that I taught a workshop called "Awakening the Glutes" for many years. One time, the day after teaching this workshop in Costa Rica, I saw a student very gingerly walking on the road. I asked if she was okay, and with the most loving snarl, she looked at me and said, "I'm so sore." This was a classic case of someone having underactive glutes and being put in a situation where they were repeatedly asked to engage them.

The gluteus medius and gluteus minimus lie on the side of the hip and are mainly responsible for abduction and internal rotation. Patients with lower back pain tend to show reduced strength and more trigger points in these muscles as opposed to those without low back pain.[9]

As part of the core, in addition to the above-mentioned, we must also consider the psoas and quadratus lumborum.

The psoas is one of the primary hip flexors and spinal stabilizers. It originates from the transverse process of T12–L4 (yes, five vertebrae in total) as well as the lateral aspects of the discs between them, and runs all the way down to the lesser trochanter of the hip. You can imagine the dysfunction that arises when this muscle is not working properly.

Despite popular belief, stretching the psoas will not cure everything from your back ache to your marital problems. The psoas actually has a tendency towards neurological inhibition, which will increase the more we stretch it. This inhibition is partially due to the flexed position we are in when sitting. This causes the psoas to become short and weak. At times, stretching it can be very beneficial, but this must be coupled with strengthening it. The combination of the two leads to more spinal stability.

The quadratus lumborum (QL) is a back muscle that originates at the posterior border of the iliac crest and inserts on the transverse process of L5–L1 and the medial border of the 12th, floating, rib. Due to its attachments, combined with that of the psoas, these two muscles are often paired in dysfunctional relationships, with one being overactive while the other is underactive.

The QL, when used unilaterally, is a lateral flexor of the spine. It is also known as the "hip hiker," and when one is stronger than the other, it creates an imbalance where one side of the pelvis is higher than the other. This leads to a functional scoliosis (quite correctable as opposed to a structural scoliosis, which is predominantly skeletal and requires a significantly larger amount of attention to fix) and weaker gluteal muscles.

The combination of all these muscles—rectus abdominus, transversus abdominus, internal/external obliques, gluteus maximus, gluteus medius, gluteus minimus, multifidus, erector spinae, hamstrings, psoas, quadratus lumborum, and let's add the quadricep muscles—should all be considered and addressed when talking about the core and working with someone who has lower back pain.

Before we begin with the practice, let's dispel another myth and get clear on the difference between an anterior pelvic tilt and a posterior pelvic tuck. An anterior tilt is one where the top of the pelvis tilts forward and the tailbone tilts backwards and up, as in Figure 4.1a. A posterior pelvic tuck (Figure 4.1b) is where the top of the buttocks moves downwards, the top of the pelvis moves backwards, and the tailbone moves forward.

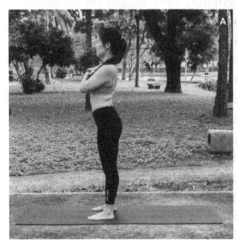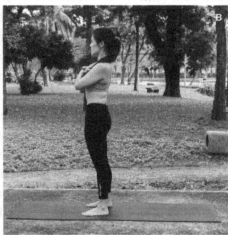

FIGURE 4.1A, B

Excessive anterior tilting of the pelvis creates a greater amount of hyperlordosis in the lumbar spine and can be a key factor in back pain. Posterior tucking of the pelvis lengthens the lower back and allows for greater abdominal and gluteus maximus activation.

This does not mean, however, that we should *always* be in a posterior tuck and that an anterior tilt is wrong. This is a huge misconception in the yoga, physical therapy, and rehabilitation training worlds. If we are always putting ourselves into a posterior tuck while shunning the anterior, the muscles of the lower back decrease their capacity to activate and the spine loses stability. It's for this reason that I have been teaching anterior tilts of the pelvis to my patients for years. Almost everyone I have worked with over the last 20 years with back pain has weak lower back muscles. This must be corrected and the following sequence is aimed at doing so.

To be clear, posterior tucks are also great. They create traction in the lower back and are taught in weeks 3 and 4 to lengthen the spine. You will also find that when we do donkey kicks in the third and fourth weeks to strengthen the glutes, I ask you to put a small grip into the lower abdomen to prevent excessive anterior tilting. The key ingredient, as you may have already inferred, is to create strength on all planes of motion, exploring those areas we are commonly told to avoid.

The following sequences are broken up into two parts. Part I is to be done for the first two weeks and Part II is for the second two weeks. You will see that some of the poses are repeated through the entire process. That is because of their ability to strengthen the muscles of the back and their proven long-term effectiveness. If at any point you feel that a pose is not helping, feel free to disregard it. Similarly, if a pose is effective for you and not in a particular sequence, you may put it in. You are the boss of your practice and know what is best for you.

Low Back Sequence Part I: Weeks 1 and 2
1. Hip hinge/chair pose

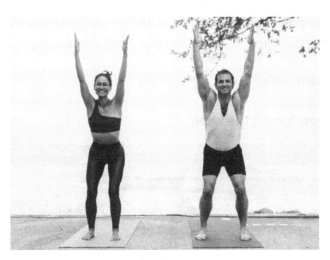

FIGURE 4.2

a. Stand with feet hip-width apart. Bend the knees and take the hips backwards. Place weight on the heels but not so much that the toes lift. Keep the pelvis in an anterior tilt (unless you have a compression-like pain and nerve referral when doing so). Take the arms over the head with the elbows straight. Lengthen the neck. Hold for five breaths. Stand up. Repeat this three times.

2. Quadratus lumborum stretch on the chair

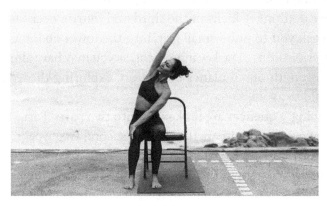

FIGURE 4.3

a. Sit on a chair with your right buttock and sit bone off the chair. Reach the left hand to the opposite knee and bend the elbow. Take the right arm above the head. Allow the right buttock to drop towards the floor as you reach the arm further above the head. You are stretching the right QL.

    -   The key to this pose is finding the position that works for you. You can pull the right knee and twist the spine more or find another way that accesses the place in your right lower back that needs it.

    Repeat two times each side.

3. Psoas stretch with the chair

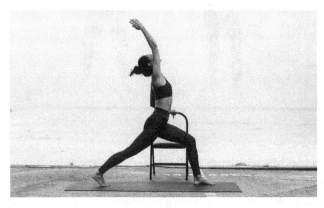

FIGURE 4.4

a. Turn a chair backwards and place it at your side. Hold on to the top of the chair for stability. Step the leg closest to the chair forward, with the other leg backwards. Keep the heel of the back leg off the ground and lift the ipsilateral (same side) arm into the air. Arch your back upwards. You are stretching the psoas of the outer leg.

Hold for just ten seconds. Repeat two times each side.

4. *Salabhasana* (locust pose)—lower body

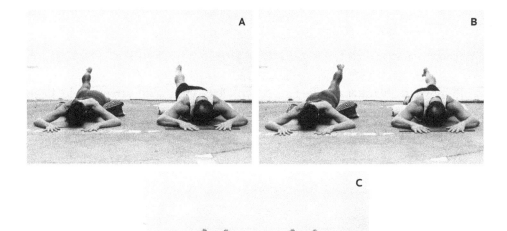

FIGURE 4.5A, B, C

a. Roll a yoga blanket lengthwise and place it directly under your anterior hip bones (anterior superior iliac spine—ASIS). This allows for a greater and more balanced lift of the leg. Take your arms overhead.

- Lift one leg. Hold for 10–20 seconds (Figure 4.5a).
- Lift the other leg (Figure 4.5b).

b. Shift forward so the blanket is now just above your pubic bone. Lift both legs (Figure 4.5c). Hold for 10–20 seconds.

Repeat three times.

5. *Salabhasana* (locust pose)—upper body

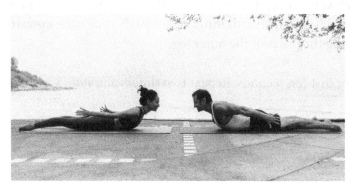

FIGURE 4.6

a. Remove the blanket and lie face down. Place your arms at your side. Keep your legs on the ground and lift the upper body, head, and arms. Hold for ten seconds. Repeat three times.

6. Bird dog

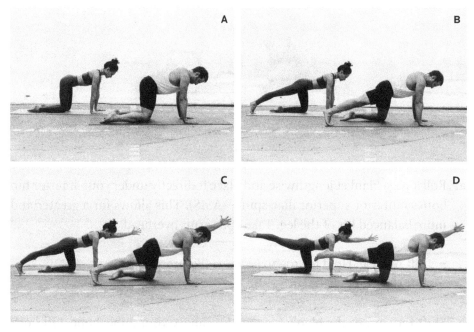

FIGURE 4.7A, B, C, D

a. Assume quadruped position with shoulders over wrists and hips over knees. Point the feet backwards with the toenails on the ground.

b. Straighten the right leg behind you and place the toe pads on the ground. Take five deep breaths into your ribs. This position allows your breath to deepen.

c. Keep the back leg on the ground and lift the opposite arm. Tighten the kneecap and elbow. Take five more breaths, this time breathing specifically into the side of the ribs of the lifted arm. On the exhalation, intentionally contract the abdomen and pull the belly button towards the spine. This helps strengthen the transverse and rectus abdominus, as well as the external oblique.

d. Full pose: Lift the leg off the ground. Keep the kneecap tight and the elbow straight. There will be some tension in your abdomen the entire time. Take five breaths, pulling the belly button towards the spine upon each exhalation.

Repeat this sequence two times on each side.

7. Myofascial release with ball

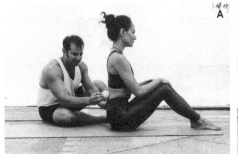 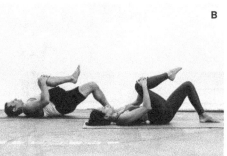

FIGURE 4.8A, B

a. Using a lacrosse, tennis, racquet, or Yoga Tune Up ball, lie on the floor with the ball just to the side of the spine, possibly on a point that has pain. Bend the knee of the opposite leg and place the foot on the floor to help give you leverage. Pull and hold the knee of the affected side towards the chest to accentuate the pressure of the ball on the lower back muscles. Look for points of pain and either hold still on them or roll side to side. Do this for 1–3 minutes, massaging anywhere that has pain.

8. *Savasana* (corpse pose)

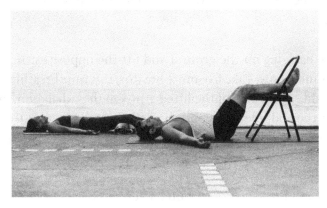

FIGURE 4.9

a. Take savasana, either with your calves on a chair or with a rolled blanket under your knees. Stay for 3–10 minutes.

Low Back Sequence Part II: Weeks 3 and 4
1. Spinal traction from *urdvha hastasana* (hands-in-the-air pose)

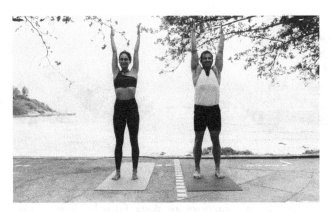

FIGURE 4.10

a. Stand with the feet hip-width apart. Take the arms over the head with palms facing each other. Press your tailbone forward and engage the glutes. Lift the ribs upwards. You should feel as though space is being created in your back body between the lower ribs and hips. Continue to work to lengthen the spine. Hold for 15–20 seconds. Inhalations will be into the ribs while the exhalations will be in the lower abdominals.

2. Hip hinge/chair pose

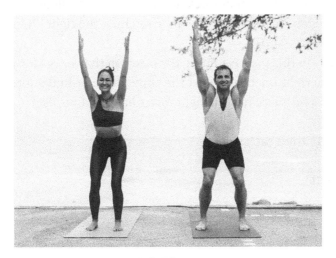

FIGURE 4.11

a. Stand with the feet hip-width apart. Bend the knees and take the hips backwards. Place weight on the heels but not so much that the toes lift. Keep the pelvis in an anterior tilt (unless you have a compression-like pain and nerve referral when doing so). Take the arms over the head with the elbows straight. Lengthen the neck. Hold for five breaths.

Stand up. Repeat this three times.

3. Quadratus lumborum stretch on the chair

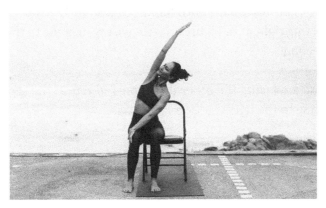

FIGURE 4.12

a. Sit on a chair with your right buttock and sit bone off the chair. Reach the left hand to the opposite knee and bend the elbow. Take the right arm above the head. Allow the right buttock to drop towards the floor as you reach the arm further above the head. You are stretching the right QL.

- The key to this pose is finding the position that works for you. You can pull the right knee and twist the spine more or find another way that accesses the place in your right lower back that needs it.

Repeat two times each side.

4. Chair twist

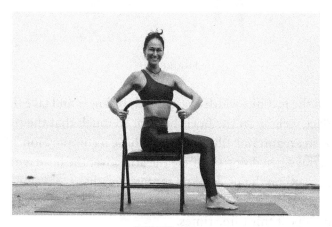

FIGURE 4.13

a. Sit sideways on the chair with both feet evenly placed on the ground. Grab hold of the chair back with both hands. Pull slightly with your left hand (when twisting right as in Figure 4.13) to twist your spine to the right. Hold for 5-10 seconds.

b. Turn so you are facing the other direction and repeat the same pose, this time twisting to the left.

Repeat three times on each side.

5. *Salabhasana* (locust pose)—lower body

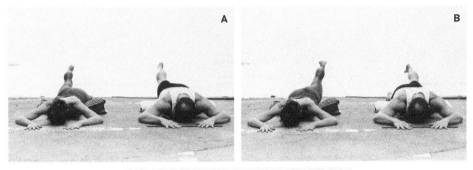

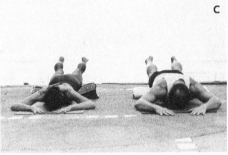

FIGURE 4.14A, B, C

a. Roll a yoga blanket lengthwise and place it directly under your anterior hip bones (ASIS). This allows for a greater and more balanced lift of the leg. Take your arms overhead.

- Lift one leg. Hold for 10–20 seconds (Figure 4.14a).
- Lift the other leg (Figure 4.14b).

b. Shift forward so the blanket is now just above your pubic bone. Lift both legs (Figure 4.14c). Hold for 10–20 seconds.

Repeat three times.

6. Prone low back traction

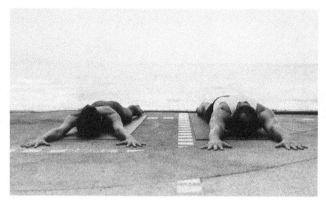

FIGURE 4.15

a. Lie face down and reach your arms over your head. Press your pubic bone down to engage the glutes. Keep the glutes engaged the whole time and take five breaths into your abdomen.

Repeat two times.

7. Bird dog

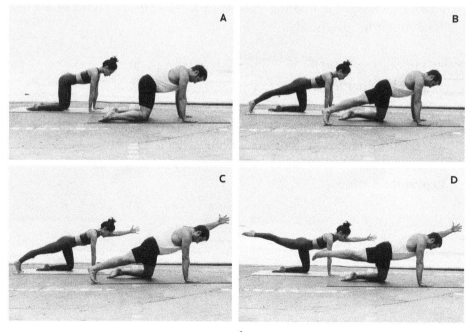

FIGURE 4.16A, B, C, D

a. Assume quadruped position with shoulders over wrists and hips over knees. Point the feet backwards with the toenails on the ground.

b. Straighten the right leg behind you and place the toe pads on the ground. Take five deep breaths into your ribs. This position allows your breath to deepen.

c. Keep the back leg on the ground and lift the opposite arm. Tighten the kneecap and elbow. Take five more breaths, this time breathing specifically into the side of the ribs of the lifted arm. On the exhalation, intentionally contract the abdomen and pull the belly button towards the spine. This helps strengthen the transverse and rectus abdominus, as well as the external oblique.

d. Full pose: Lift the leg off the ground. Keep the kneecap tight and the elbow straight. There will be some tension in your abdomen the entire time. Take five breaths, pulling the belly button towards the spine upon each exhalation. Repeat this sequence two times on each side.

8. Donkey kicks

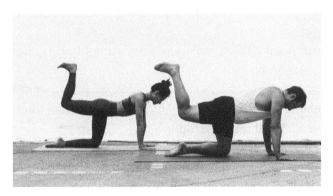

FIGURE 4.17

a. Assume the quadruped position. Place a small grip into the lower abdomen to prevent the lumbar spine from overarching. With the knee bent, lift one leg into the air and then lower it back down. Repeat this 5–8 times. On the eighth repetition, hold the position in the air and lift the leg a little higher, attaining maximum activation of the gluteus maximus. Remember to always keep the small grip in the lower abdomen and prevent overarching (hyperlordosis) of the lumbar spine.

Repeat three times on each side.

9. Plank variations

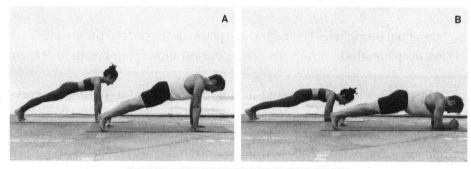

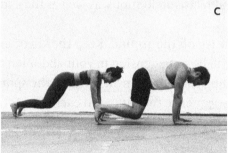

FIGURE 4.18A, B, C

a. Straight arm plank: Take plank pose with straight arms and straight legs. Hold for 20 seconds.

b. Forearm plank: Assume forearm plank with the fingers interlaced and the elbows spread. Hold for 20 seconds.

c. Quadruped plank: From quadruped, lift the knees off ground. Hold for five breaths. Let the breath guide your alignment in this pose. It will show you where your pelvis is twisted or your shoulders are misaligned. Make the appropriate adjustments.

- **Note:** For the straight arm and forearm plank: The pelvis can be neutral, slightly anterior or in a posterior tuck. The posterior tuck will engage the transversus abdominus more than in the other positions. Feel free to explore the position that feels like it's the most effective for you.

Repeat each variation two times.

10. Myofascial release with ball

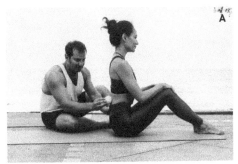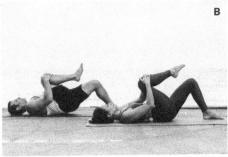

FIGURE 4.19

a. Using a lacrosse, tennis, racquet, or Yoga Tune Up ball, lie on the floor with the ball just to the side of the spine, possibly on the point that has pain. Bend the knee of the opposite leg and place the foot on the floor to help give you leverage. Pull and hold the knee of the affected side towards the chest to accentuate the pressure of the ball on the lower back muscles. Look for points of pain and either hold still on them or roll side to side. Do this for 1–3 minutes, massaging anywhere that has pain.

11. *Savasana* (corpse pose)

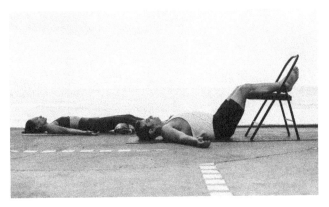

FIGURE 4.20

a. Take *savasana*, either with your calves on a chair or with a rolled blanket under your knees. Stay for 3–10 minutes.

CHAPTER 5

Anatomy of the Hip

The hip, like the shoulder, is a ball-and-socket joint. Its purpose is to support the weight of the body when standing, walking, or running. It also transfers strength from the lower limbs into the torso.

The hip joint consists of the head of the femur, which fits into a circular cavity in the pelvis called the acetabulum. Holding it in place is the joint capsule and four very strong ligaments. Surrounding the hip are 19 different muscles: the three glutes, five adductors, six external rotators, and five main hip flexors.

Due to a lack of attention on maintaining strength and ranges of motion, the hip tends to degenerate the older we get. According to the Agency of Healthcare Research and Quality, there are around 450,000 hip replacements performed every year in the United States (1 person in 738 has a hip replacement per year).[1] We can compare that to around 59,000 per year in Japan (1 person in 2131 has a hip replacement per year),[2] where people often sit on the floor cross-legged with ease until their old age.

There are seven ranges of motion the hip can experience, making it the second most mobile joint in the body, next to the shoulder. They are:

1. flexion
2. extension
3. abduction
4. adduction
5. external rotation
6. internal rotation
7. circumduction.

A limitation in any of these can lead to significant dysfunction. In most patients who do need hip replacements, internal rotation (IR) is the primary range of motion that degenerates first. Thus, having a practice of maintaining IR is crucial as we get older.

The three main muscles that internally rotate the hip are the gluteus medius, gluteus minimus, and tensor fascia latae. Gluteus medius dysfunction has been linked to everything from hip to low back to knee and neck pain. Decreased neuromuscular muscle activity here will cause adduction of the hip joint during weight bearing and walking. This will increase the Q-angle and valgus of the femur, thus putting more stress on the hip and knee.[3]

As reported by Distefano *et al.*,[4] side-lying hip abductions have a significantly greater activity on the gluteus medius than the even more popular clamshell exercise. Thus, they should be practiced in any hip, knee, or lower back dysfunction.

Throughout this sequence, we will target both flexibility and strength. The overly taut adductors and external rotators will be stretched while the commonly weaker areas such as the abductors and psoas will be strengthened.

In addition, we will also use something called a CAR to create articular health. CAR stands for controlled articular rotation and comes from the Functional Anatomy Seminars team. It is not just a simple rotation or joint circle that was taught in 1980s aerobic classes but a more intentional movement that reaches and maintains control through the outer ranges of a joint. This requires a greater amount of motor control and concentration than most people are used to. It generates strength in muscle fibers that are often inactive and creates mobility in areas that are commonly stuck. Hip CARS will be introduced in the third week of this program but the same principles of strength and control should be applied to the *supine hip circles* in week 1 and 2.

ANATOMY OF THE HIP   121

Hip Sequence Part I: Weeks 1 and 2
1. *Supta padangusthasana I, II, II* (reclining hand-to-big-toe pose)

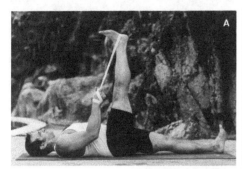
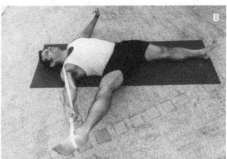
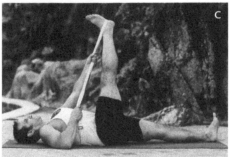

FIGURE 5.1A, B, C

a. Hook a strap around the foot and bring the leg into the air towards the ceiling (Figure 5.1a). Hold for one minute.

b. Shorten the outer side of the strap and hold both sides of it with your outer arm. Take the strap behind your head and hold it with the opposite hand. Take the leg out to the side (Figure 5.1b). Hold for 30 seconds.

c. Bring the leg back up to the ceiling and move it across the body to the opposite side. *Keep the sacrum on the floor.* The leg will only go a few inches and that's okay! Hold for 15–30 seconds (Figure 5.1c).

You only need to do each of these once on each side.

2. Figure 4

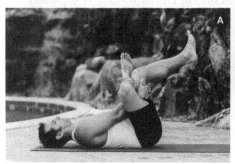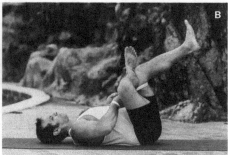

FIGURE 5.2A, B

a. Lie on your back with both knees bent. Cross one ankle over the top of the opposite knee. Bring the legs into the air and grab behind the knee. Keep that knee around a 110° angle (Figure 5.2a). This aids in the stretch. Hold for 10–20 seconds.

b. If you cannot reach behind your knee, hook a strap around it and hold that (Figure 5.2b).

Repeat three times on each side .

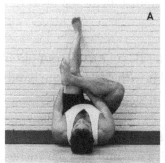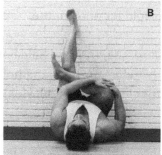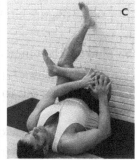

FIGURE 5.3A, B, C

Bonus (Figure 5.3a, b, c): If practicing where you have access to a wall, lie with your legs up the wall and cross one ankle over the opposite knee. Grab behind the straight leg and bend it (while keeping the heel on the wall) until you get a stretch in the opposite hip (Figure 5.3a).

- Pull the bent knee closer to your chest (Figure 5.3b).
- Push the bent knee away from your chest (Figure 5.3c).

3. Supine hip circles with straight leg

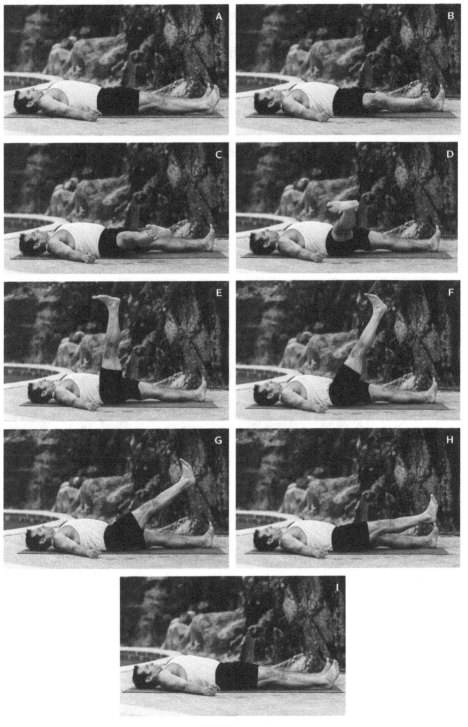

FIGURE 5.4A-1

a. Lie on the floor with your arms at your sides. Make fists with your hands and press them down into the floor to create stability. Lift one leg into the air and perform a full circle with the leg. *Keep the opposite leg straight and active. Do not let the pelvis rotate. The sacrum should stay in contact with the floor at all times.* Attempt to reach the outer ranges of motion with the hip joint of the moving leg.

- Do four circles in each direction.

Important note: There will be places of weakness through this circle that your body will want to skip over. At these exact spots, pause and see if you can hold them. This will increase the motor unit development and strength in the area.

4. Goddess pose

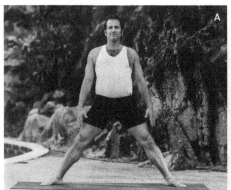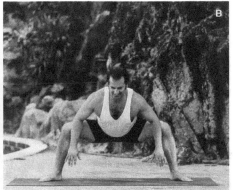

FIGURE 5.5A, B

a. Stand with your legs 3–4 feet apart with the feet turned outwards. Squat down and place your forearm just above the inner knee. Press the inner knees outwards, creating a strong stretch in the adductors. Hold for 10–20 seconds, increasing the stretch the longer you hold it for.

Repeat two times.

5. Side-lying abduction

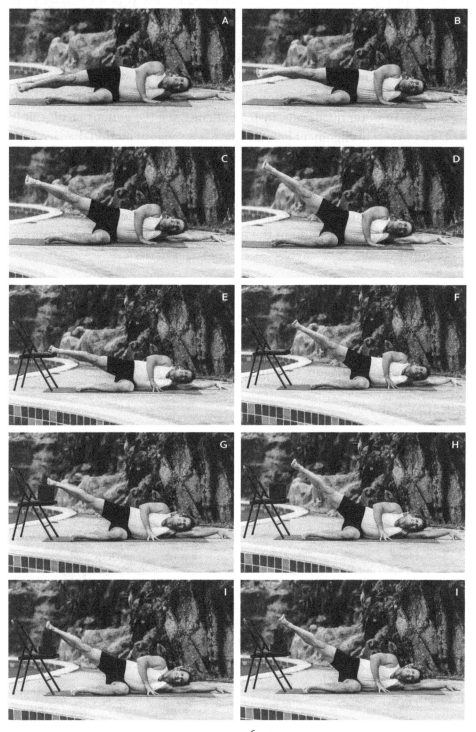

FIGURE 5.6A–J

a. Lie on your side with your ear, shoulder, hip, and ankle in one straight line. Bend the bottom knee to 90° in front of you. Place your arm under your head for support.

b. Lift your top leg into the air, keeping the ankle and hip in line with the shoulder. Do not let your pelvis roll backwards or allow your hip to externally rotate. These are common cheats and cause you to use the low back muscles or outer quadriceps instead of engaging the gluteus medius. It is better to stay in alignment here and have less range of motion than to cheat and have "more" range. Repeat lifting and lowering the leg five times.

On the fifth repetition, hold the leg in its maximum range of motion for ten seconds and see if you can then lift it a little higher. Keep looking for more muscular activation in the hip socket and greater range of motion (Figure 5.6a–d).

- Variations of this include placing your foot on a chair and lifting it off from there. As you can see in the pictures, depending on your strength and range of motion, you can even prop the chair up higher with blocks. The key is being honest with your range of motion capacities and *not compensating* (Figure 5.6d–j).

6. Happy baby

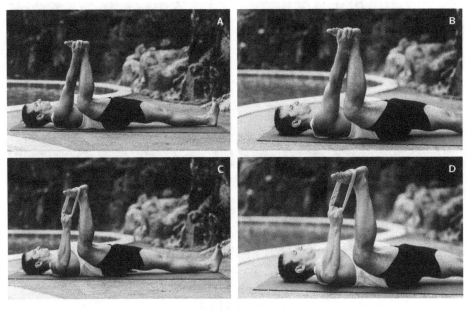

FIGURE 5.7A–D

a. Lie on your back. Bend the knee, reach through the anterior portion of the shin and grab hold of the pinky side of the foot. Pull the knee towards the floor. Make sure the shin is perpendicular to the floor. Straighten your elbow and pull the back of your shoulder towards the floor (Figure 5.7a, b).

- If you cannot grab your foot, use a strap (Figure 5.7c, d).

Repeat two times per side.

7. Myofascial release with a ball

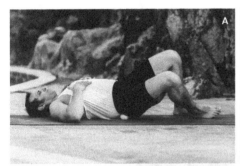
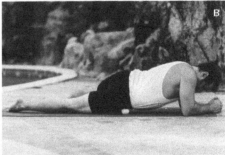
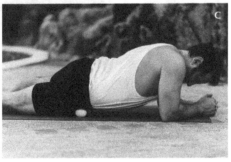

FIGURE 5.8A–C

a. Lie on your back with the knees bent and place a ball underneath your buttocks. Roll around on the ball, searching for the tighter, more sensitive areas. When you find one, stay there for a bit before moving to the next spot (Figure 5.8a).

- Most of us only roll the gluteus maximus, gluteus medius, and gluteus minimus when rolling out our hips but the tensor fascia latae (TFL) is just as important. The TFL is an anterolateral muscle of the hip that originates at the ASIS and inserts distally to the iliotibial band. (Yes, the

IT band is pretty much the tendon for the TFL.) To roll the TFL, place the ball directly on it and lie face down, propped up on your elbows. Find the spot in the anterior hip, just distal to the ASIS, that feels super sensitive. That's it. Roll around on here and pause when you find an area of pain (Figure 5.8a, b, c).

Hip Sequence Part II: Weeks 3 and 4

1. *Supta padangusthasana I, II, II* (reclining hand-to-toe pose)

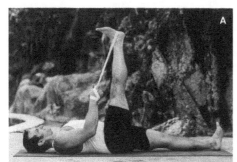
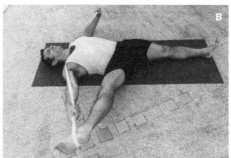
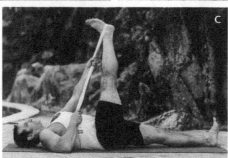

FIGURE 5.9A–C

a. Hook a strap around the foot and bring the leg into the air towards the ceiling (Figure 5.9a). Hold for one minute.

b. Shorten the outer side of the strap and hold both sides of it with your outer arm. Take the strap behind your head and hold it with the opposite hand. Take the leg out to the side (Figure 5.9b). Hold for 30 seconds.

c. Bring the leg back up to the ceiling and move it across the body to the opposite side (Figure 5.9c). *Keep the sacrum on the floor.* The leg will only go a few inches and that's okay! Hold for 15–30 seconds.

You only need to do each of these once.

ANATOMY OF THE HIP 129

2. Supine hip circles with straight leg

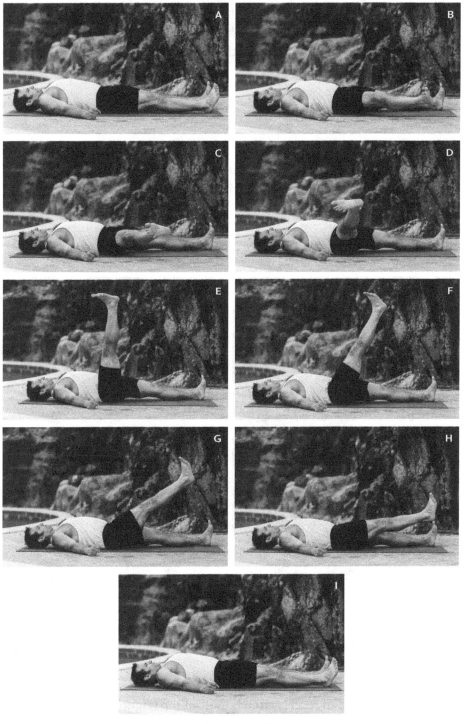

FIGURE 5.10A–1

a. Lie on the floor with your arms at your sides. Make fists with your hands and press them down into the floor to create stability. Lift one leg into the air and perform a full circle with the leg. *Keep the opposite leg straight and active. Do not let the pelvis rotate. The sacrum should stay in contact with the floor at all times.* Attempt to reach the outer ranges of motion with the hip joint of the moving leg.

b. Do four circles in each direction.

   - **Important note:** There will be places of weakness through this circle that your body will want to skip over. At these exact spots, pause and see if you can hold them. This will increase the motor unit development and strength in the area.

3. 90/90

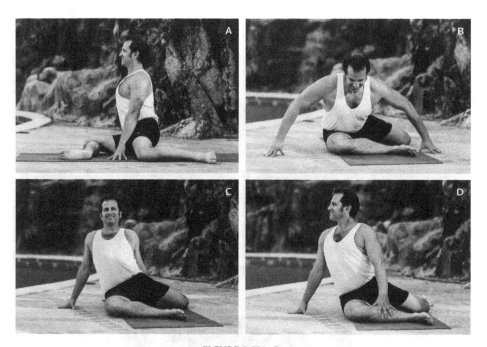

FIGURE 5.11A–D

a. Sit on the ground and create a 90° angle with your front hip/knee/shin and back hip/knee/shin (Figure 5.11a).

   - Lean forward to receive stretch in front hip (Figure 5.11b).

- Sit up tall and place hands on floor. Sensation should be felt in the anterior portion of the back hip. Lean backward slightly to increase stretch and internal rotation (Figure 5.11c).
- Twist upright over the front leg five times while squeezing the opposite glute (Figure 5.11d).

Repeat two times on each side.

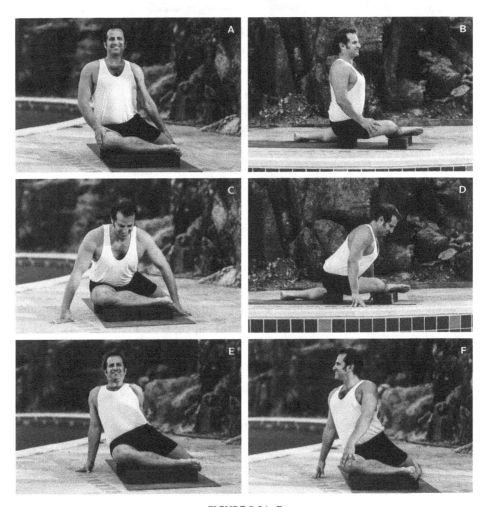

FIGURE 5.2A–F

Variation with blocks: If you are unable or uncomfortable sitting on the floor in this 90/90 position, elevate yourself on three blocks. If your right leg is forward, one block goes under your right buttock and two blocks go under the right shin. Your left knee will be on the ground (Figure 5.12).

4. Groin release with block

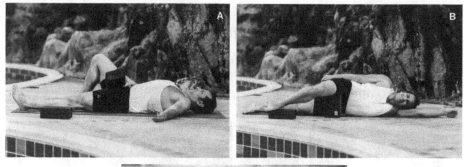

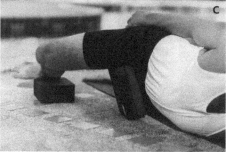

FIGURE 5.13A–C

a. Lie on your back and place one block to the left of you, around the level of the shin. Bend the right knee and place the other block the long way up against your groin, near the attachment on the pubis (Figure 5.13a). Roll to the left side so the block on your groin is upright and your foot is resting on the other block (Figure 5.13b, c). This prevents your hip from going into external rotation and allows you to feel the massage. Rest here for 1–2 minutes.

b. To increase the pressure, lean left a little more to cause the bottom edge of the block to tip upwards. This will also pressurize the upper portion of the block against your adductor longus tendon. Enjoy!

5. Side-lying abduction

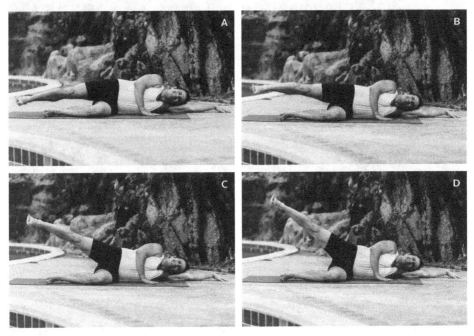

FIGURE 5.14A–D

a. Lie on your side with your ear, shoulder, hip, and ankle in one straight line. Bend the bottom knee to 90° in front of you. Place your arm under your head for support.

b. Lift your top leg into the air, keeping the ankle and hip in line with the shoulder. Do not let your pelvis roll backwards or allow your hip to externally rotate. These are common cheats and cause you to use the low back muscles or outer quadriceps instead of engaging the gluteus medius. It is better to stay in alignment here and have less range of motion than to cheat and have "more" range. Repeat lifting and lowering the leg five times.

- On the fifth repetition, hold the leg in its maximum range of motion for ten seconds and see if you can then lift it a little higher. Keep looking for more muscular activation in the hip socket and greater range of motion (Figure 5.14a–d)

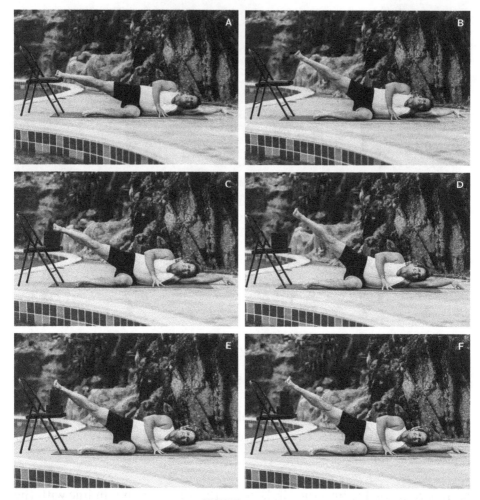

FIGURE 5.15A–F

Variations of this include placing your foot on a chair and lifting it off from there. As you can see in the pictures, depending on your strength and range of motion, you can even prop the chair up higher with blocks. The key is being honest with your range of motion capacities and *not compensating* (Figures 5.15).

6. Hip CARS

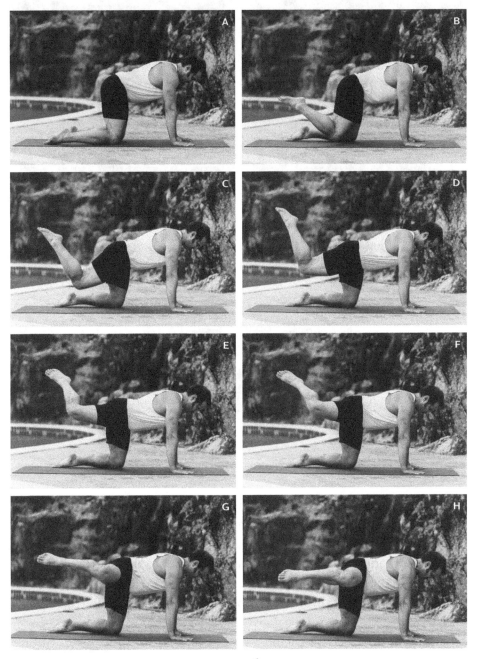

FIGURE 5.16A–H

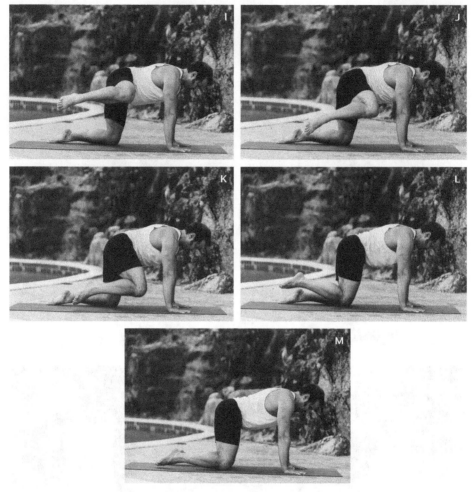

FIGURE 5.161-M

a. Assume the quadruped position with your shoulders over wrists and hips directly above your knees. Put a small grip into the lower abdomen. Lift one leg behind you with the knee bent and without arching your back. Make a circular motion with your hip by bringing it out to the side. Work hard to maintain the full height of the hip. Bring it forward and back down to the ground. This is one revolution. Repeat this four times in each direction.

Common cheats in this will be:

- bending the elbows
- shooting the hips off to the side
- overly rotating the spine.

Try not to do these! You can put your non-moving hip up against a wall to help you not compensate. This is a difficult action! It's better not to cheat and have less range than to cheat and have a lot of range.

7. Myofascial release with a ball

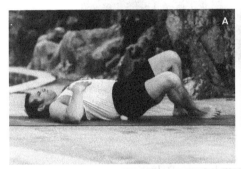
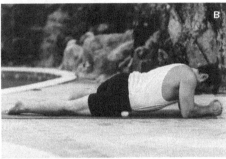
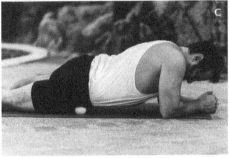

FIGURE 5.17A–C

a. Lie on your back with the knees bent and place a ball underneath your buttocks. Roll around on the ball, searching for the tighter, more sensitive areas. When you find one, stay there for a bit before moving to the next spot (Figure 5.17a).

- Most of us only roll the gluteus maximus, gluteus medius, and gluteus minimus when rolling out our hips but the tensor fascia latae (TFL) is just as important. The TFL is an anterolateral muscle of the hip that originates at the ASIS and inserts distally to the iliotibial band. (Yes, the IT band is pretty much the tendon for the TFL.) To roll the TFL, place the ball directly on it and lie face down, propped up on your elbows. Find the spot in the anterior hip, just distal to the ASIS, that feels super sensitive. That's it. Roll around on here and pause when you find an area of pain (Figure 5.8a, b, c).

8. *Savasana* (corpse pose) with bolster under knees

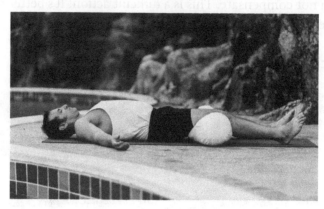

FIGURE 5.18

a. Lie supine with a bolster under your knees. Palms are face up about 25° away from your body. Rest for 3–10 minutes.

CHAPTER 6

Anatomy of the Knee

The knee is a modified hinge joint. This means that it has the ability to flex and extend (like a normal hinge) but also has rotational qualities (your shin should be able to turn slightly in and out).

There are three bones that comprise the knee: the femur, the tibia, and the patella. Holding these three bones together are four ligaments. They are the anterior cruciate ligament (ACL), posterior cruciate ligament (PCL), medial collateral ligament (MCL), and lateral collateral ligament (LCL).

The three hamstring muscles on the back of your thigh (biceps femoris, semimembranosus, and semitendinosus) all attach on different parts of the posterior tibia and fibula. They are responsible for bending your knee and extending your hip. The four quadricep muscles on the front of your thigh (rectus femoris, vastus lateralis, vastus medialis, and vastus intermedius) all attach on the anterior portion of your tibia at the tibial tuberosity via the patella tendon. These muscles are responsible for extending (straightening) your knee and flexing your hip.

In between the femur and tibia are crescent-shaped cartilage discs called meniscus. These are shock absorbers and reduce the friction inside the knee when it moves from flexion to extension. Meniscal tears are common injuries yet many are asymptomatic and the effectiveness of meniscus surgery is heavily debated. Many meniscus injuries heal on their own, either with time or from a physical therapy/yoga therapy approach. Creating balance of the muscles around the knee brings back stability and mobility to the joint.

As people get older, they also tend to lose their ability to flex the knee. The child who sits on the floor in between her shins with her knees bent is rarely doing the same thing at 50. We want to maintain the flexion (and extension) of the knee as we get older. To do this, we practice both flexion and extension. A teacher I know once said, "You know what the 80-year-old woman who's still doing splits to this day did to be able to achieve that? Splits!"

A healthy knee has four main components:

1. the ability to flex properly
2. the ability to fully extend
3. muscular balance around the joint
4. the ability to bear weight during varying levels of knee flexion.

Numbers 1 and 2 can be done passively and don't necessarily demand strength, but 3 and 4 do require strength.

Muscular balance around the joint means that the hamstrings, quadriceps, adductors, and abductors all maintain function, strength, and flexibility. When the hamstrings get overly taut, they pull the knee into flexion and inhibit the quadriceps. When the adductors get tight, they increase the Q-angle from the hip to the knee and weaken the abductors.

In many cases of knee pain, the vastus medialis obliquus (VMO) is weak and undeveloped. The VMO locks the knee and provides stability to the kneecap and medial meniscus. When it becomes weak, the kneecap tends to shift laterally. A weak VMO is often coupled with an excessively tight popliteus. The popliteus is an antagonistic muscle to the VMO and unlocks the knee during the first ten degrees of flexion. It originates at the lateral femoral condyle and lateral meniscus, crosses the back of the knee, and attaches to the medial tibia. Popliteus injuries often mimic symptoms of meniscal tears. Because the popliteus is so small and strong, it has even been considered the fifth ligament of the knee. Releasing the popliteus while strengthening the VMO is a common recipe for success and part of the knee program that follows.

Contrasting this pattern would be someone who is "quad dominant." This is a situation where the quadriceps are overdeveloped and the hamstrings are weak. This can be seen in cyclists with overdeveloped quads. It's also quite often seen in yogis who are always stretching their hamstrings and doing very little to strengthen them.

The ability to weight bear during varying levels of flexion is the key ingredient to being able to walk up and down hills and stairs and to jog. It is possibly the most important of the "four healthy knee components" in terms of health and longevity. When people squat or take chair pose (*utkatasana*), they are challenging the strength of the knees in flexion. Squats significantly strengthen the glutes and quadriceps, both components of functional knee activity.

MYTH BUST # 6

YOUR KNEES SHOULD NEVER GO PAST YOUR TOES

One of the biggest myths in the knee world is that the knees should never go past the toes. This goes back to the "alignment or nothing" regime and goes against the body's need for variability. Whether it's a lunge, a squat, or even *virabhadrasana II* (warrior II), the common thought is that this will be damaging.

It appears this myth began in 1978 after a Duke University study showed that the knees experienced less shearing forces during a squat when the shin was held in a vertical position as opposed to gliding past the toes. The problem with this is exactly what we spoke of earlier: if you have a range of motion available and avoid using it, the moment your body unintentionally goes into that position you are at risk of injury because you haven't trained the muscles to react accordingly.

Our knees go past our toes in a multitude of positions, including going down stairs, bicycling, lunges, sprinting, and squats. By training these positions, we significantly strengthen our knee joints and reduce the risk of injury. In fact, concerns about degenerative changes in the knee such as chondromalacia and osteoarthritis from deeps squats is completely unfounded.[1]

By consciously allowing the knee to go past the toes, we also develop more ankle dorsiflexion. This has continually been shown to positively affect knee health.[2] By creating a healthy range of motion in one joint, we positively affect the joints above and below it. If we limit the range of motion in one joint, the others will have to make shifts to accommodate this lack of mobility.

The following is a four-week sequence to help almost anyone with knee pain. It is recommended to do this sequence at least four times a week to gain the greatest advantage.

Knee Sequence Part I: Weeks 1 and 2

1. *Supta padangusthasana I* (reclining hand-to-big-toe pose) with a strap

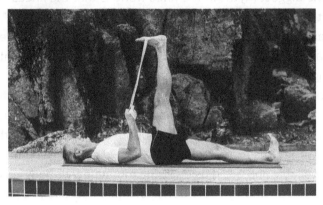

FIGURE 6.1

a. Hook a strap around the metatarsals. Keep the knee completely straight. It does not matter how high your leg goes. Pull the strap to get the foot into dorsiflexion and stretch the back of the knee. Hold for 30 seconds. Repeat two times on each side.

2. Downward-facing dog sequence

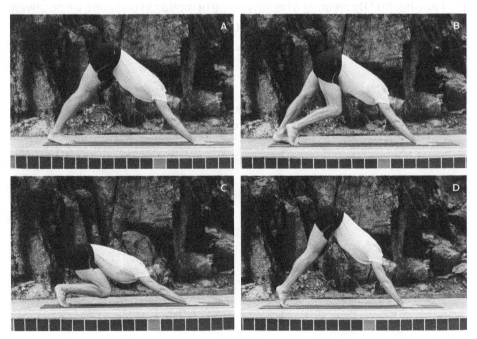

FIGURE 6.2A–D

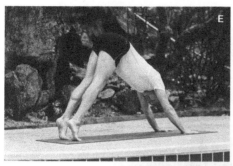
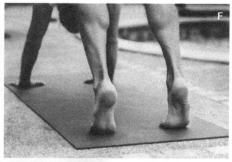
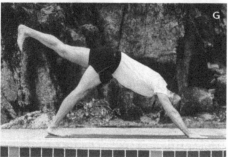

FIGURE 6.2E–G

a. Assume down dog with both knees straight (Figure 6.2a).

   - Bend one knee and press the opposite heel down (Figure 6.2b).

   - Bend both knees so they hover a few inches over the ground (Figure 6.2c). Hold for ten seconds and then straighten both legs. Repeat two times.

   - With straight knees, lift the heels so the toes get stretched. You can press the heels closer together to get a stretch in the big toes or separate them slightly to get a stretch in the other four toes (Figure 6.2d–f).

   - With straight knees, lift one leg behind you (Figure 6.2g). Grip just above the inner knee of the standing leg. This is the vastus medialis obliquus (VMO). Hold for at least ten seconds.

   Repeat two times on each side.

3. Popliteus stretch with a chair

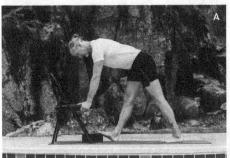
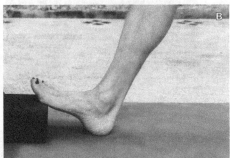

FIGURE 6.3A, B

a. Set up a chair so it won't slide. Place one block at its lowest height directly under the chair seat. Place your metatarsals of your foot on top of a block. The heel stays on the floor. Place your hands on the chair seat and step the opposite leg backwards 2–3 feet. *The foot of that leg must face directly forward.* Straighten the front leg. If there is any bend at all, this will not work. Lengthen/flatten the spine. Hold for 20–30 seconds. Repeat two times on each side.

4. *Virabhadrasana II* (warrior II)

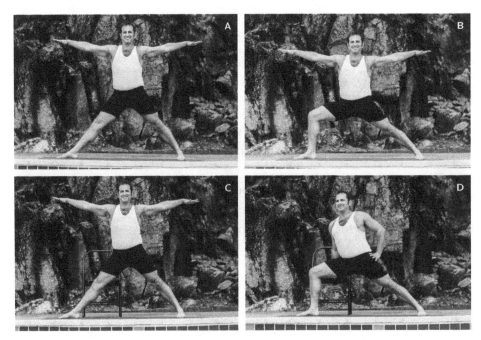

FIGURE 6.4A–D

a. Separate the feet 3½–4½ feet apart. Align the front heel with the back arch (Figure 6.4a). Bend and straighten the knee three times (Figure 6.4b). On the third time, hold for 20 seconds. Repeat two times on each side.

- If there is not enough strength to do this, place a chair behind you and your hand on the chair for support (Figure 6.4c, d).

5. Short lunge

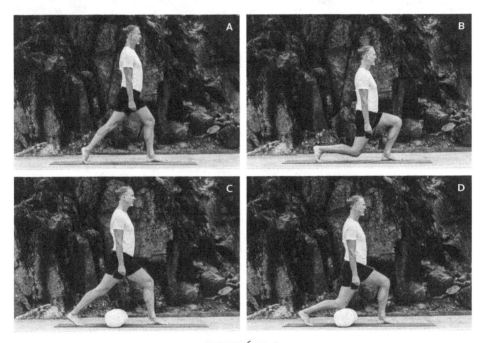

FIGURE 6.5A–D

a. Separate the feet for a short lunge (Figure 6.5a). Bend the back knee so it hovers over the floor (Figure 6.5b). Hold for five seconds then straighten both knees. Repeat five times on each side.

- If there is fear in the back knee, place a bolster underneath it for support (Figure 6.5c, d).

6. *Ushtrasana* (camel pose) lean backs

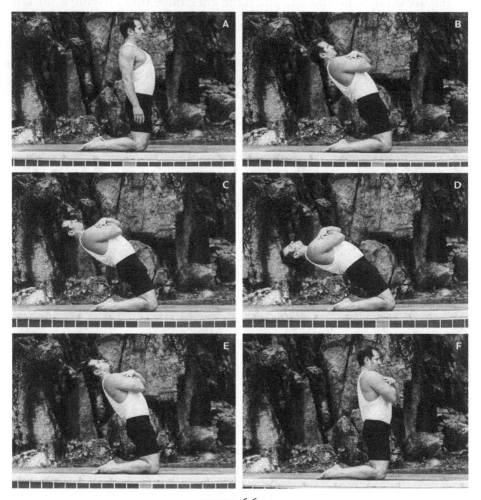

FIGURE 6.6A–F

a. Kneel on your knees and shins with the toes pointing backwards and toenails on the floor. Cross your arms at your chest and press the shins into floor. Lean the torso backwards as far as you can safely and comfortably, then come back up. Repeat 5–8 times. Try to increase your range of motion each time.

7. *Virasana* (hero's pose)

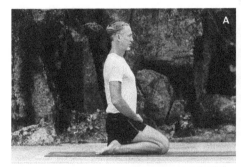
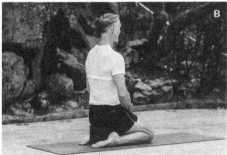
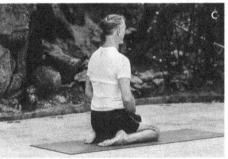

FIGURE 6.7A–C

a. Sit on a block with the heels separated and knees close together. Find the right height that allows you to hold the pose for 1–3 minutes without pain. The pictures show two blocks (Figure 6.7a, b) and one block (Figure 6.7c), but you can use four blocks if needed.

8. *Savasana* (corpse pose)

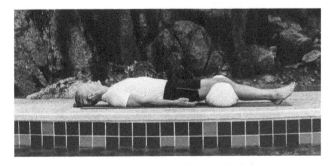

FIGURE 6.8

a. Lie on your back with a bolster under your knees, palms face up, and arms around 20–30° away from your body. Stay for 3–10 minutes.

Knee Sequence Part II: Weeks 3 and 4
1. Downward-facing dog sequence

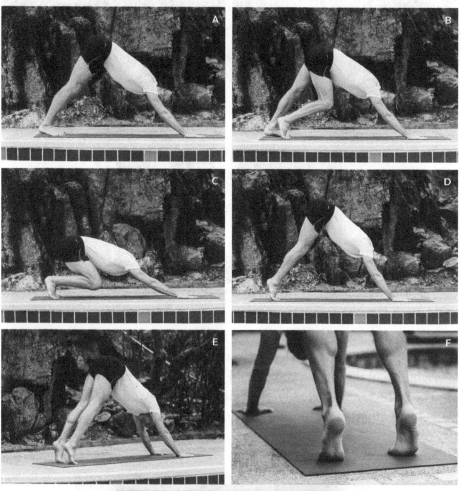

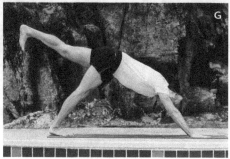

FIGURE 6.9A–G

a. Assume down dog with both knees straight (Figure 6.9a). Bend one knee and press the opposite heel down (Figure 6.9b). Bend both knees so they hover a few inches over the ground (Figure 6.9c). Hold for ten seconds and then straighten both legs. Repeat two times.

b. With straight knees, lift the heels so the toes get stretched. You can press the heels closer together to get a stretch in the big toes or separate them slightly to get a stretch in the other four toes (Figure 6.9d-f).

c. With straight knees, lift one leg behind you (Figure 6.9g). Grip just above the inner knee of the standing leg. This is the vastus medialis obliquus (VMO). Hold for at least ten seconds.

Repeat two times per side.

2. Popliteus stretch with a chair

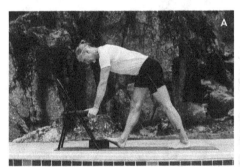
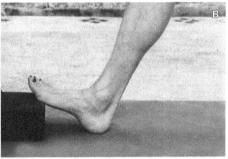

FIGURE 6.10A, B

a. Set up a chair so it won't slide. Place one block at its lowest height directly under the chair seat. Place your metatarsals of your foot on top of a block. The heel stays on the floor. Place your hands on the chair seat and step the opposite leg backwards 2-3 feet. *The foot of that leg must face directly forward.* Straighten the front leg. If there is any bend at all, this will not work. Lengthen/flatten the spine. Hold for 20-30 seconds. Repeat two times on each side.

3. Sit to stands on a chair

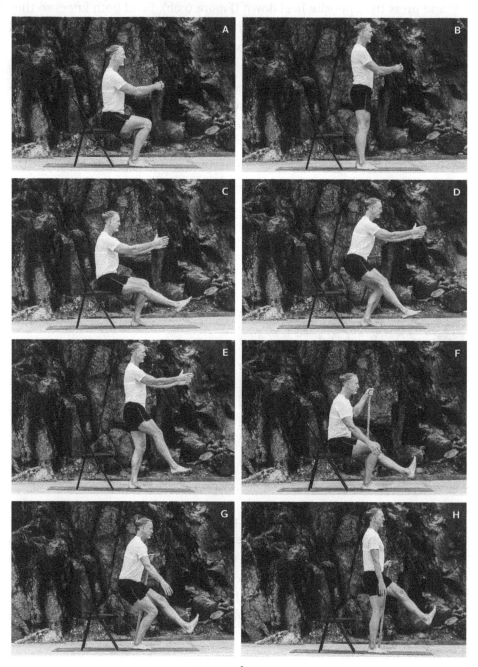

FIGURE 6.11A–H

a. Begin by practicing with both legs (Figure 6.11a, b). You should be able to stand and slowly sit back down without the use of your hands. If you cannot, continue to practice this until you develop the strength. You may also use a stick for support as in the figures.

b. One leg: Place one foot on the ground and straighten the other leg off the ground. Stand up and then sit down. Repeat 3–5 times if possible (Figure 6.11c–e).

- Look for varus/valgus in the knee and overpronation/supination in the foot.

c. If this is too difficult, hold a stick on the opposite side of the bent knee and push it downwards to aid in standing up (Figure 6.11f–h).

4. Bulgarian split squat

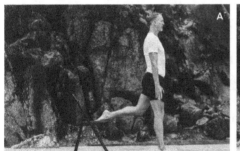
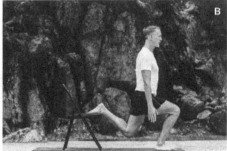
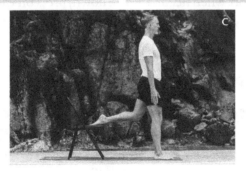

FIGURE 6.12A–C

a. Place the top of your foot on a chair with the other foot about 2–2½ feet away from the chair. Bend the front knee and straighten it. Do 5–8 repetitions and repeat two times on each side.

5. Eccentric lunge sit-backs

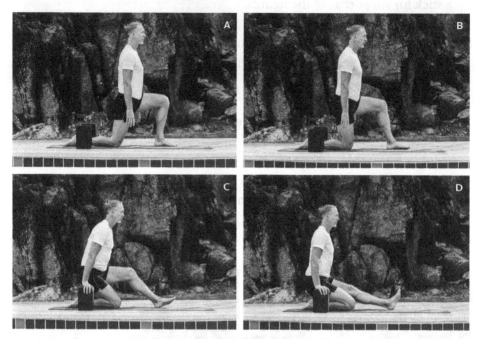

FIGURE 6.13A–D

a. Take a lunge with the back knee down and toenails on the ground. Place one block on either side of the back shin. Sit backwards slowly, using the blocks for support when needed. Once down, press off the bent knee to rise back up. Repeat 3–5 times on each side. If you feel strong enough to perform this without the blocks, feel free.

6. *Savasana* (corpse pose)

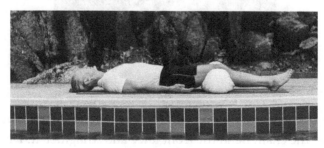

FIGURE 6.14

a. Lie on your back with a bolster under your knees, palms face up and arms around 20–30° away from your body. Stay for 3–10 minutes.

CHAPTER 7

Anatomy of the Shoulder

The shoulder is one of the most complex systems in the human body. There are four joints that comprise what is generally referred to as the shoulder girdle. They are the glenohumeral, sternoclavicular, acromioclavicular, and scapulothoracic. The glenohumeral joint, a ball-and-socket joint, is the most mobile joint in the body. Because of this, and the body's tendency to protect, there is a propensity for this joint to be either hypermobile or hypomobile.

The glenohumeral joint articulates the head of the humerus with the glenoid fossa of the scapula. There is articular cartilage lining the surfaces of each along with synovial fluid that helps to reduce friction.[1] In addition to the synovial fluid, there are four main bursae that act as a cushion between the joint structures. They are the subacromial, subdeltoid, subcoracoid, and subscapular bursa.

The humeral head is also quite large in relation to the glenoid fossa, and this contributes to it being the most commonly dislocated joint.[2] The stabilizing structures of the joint include the joint capsule (glenohumeral ligaments), coracoclavicular ligament, coracohumeral ligament, glenoid labrum, long head of the biceps (which attaches to the labrum), and rotator cuff muscles.

All of the nerves that supply the glenohumeral joint originate from the C5–T1 vertebrae and a bundle of nerves called the brachial plexus. The brachial plexus provides sensory and motor information to all the muscles of the shoulder except the trapezius. After originating in the cervical spine, it passes through the scalenes, and runs under the clavicle and pectoralis minor though the arm to terminate in the hand. Evaluation of the neck and brachial plexus is important in all shoulder problems.

The four muscles of the rotator cuff are the supraspinatus, infraspinatus, teres minor, and subscapularis. Their main job is stabilization of the glenohumeral joint by compressing the humeral head into the socket.

The supraspinatus abducts the shoulder for the initial 15 degrees. The infraspinatus and teres minor aid in external rotation while the subscapularis aids in internal rotation.

Rotator cuff injuries are the most common source of shoulder pain for primary care visits.[3] These could include anything from tendinitis, tears, subacromial bursitis, or impingement syndromes.

Similar to the hip, the shoulder has seven ranges of motions. Most of these are larger than that of the hip, however, due to the anatomical limitations presented by the depth of the acetabulum and placement of the head of the femur in the socket.

These ranges of motion are:

1. flexion
2. extension
3. abduction
4. adduction
5. external rotation
6. internal rotation
7. circumduction.

A functional shoulder joint has flexibility and strength through all of these motions.

The scapula is another important part of the shoulder, and connects the clavicle to the humerus. There are 17 muscles that attach to it: the four rotator cuff muscles, the trapezius, teres major, triceps brachii (long head), biceps brachii, rhomboid major, rhomboid minor, coracobrachialis, latissimus dorsi, deltoid, levator scapulae, pectoralis minor, serratus anterior, and inferior belly of the omohyoid.

There are four main types of motion of the scapula:

1. protraction
2. retraction
3. elevation
4. depression.

Protraction is created by the serratus anterior, pectoralis major, and pectoralis minor muscles. Retraction is achieved by the rhomboids, trapezius, and latissimus dorsi. Elevation is accomplished by the trapezius, levator scapulae, and rhomboids. Depression is performed by the latissimus dorsi, serratus anterior, pectoralis major/minor, and trapezius.

You may have noticed that the trapezius performs retraction, elevation, and depression, three opposing actions. This is because the shape of the muscle is divided into three different segments, all having different functions. Assessing a shoulder problem often asks us to differentiate which aspects of the trapezius are overactive and which are underactive.

Dysfunctions of the muscles of the scapula, particularly that of an overly taut pectoralis minor, can lead to dyskinesis, a situation where either the normal resting position or the functional movement of the scapula is significantly altered. In the case of a winged scapula, where paralysis of the serratus anterior or trapezius may occur, the ability to achieve full flexion of the glenohumeral joint is severely limited.[4]

The following sequence is aimed at increasing the range of motion and strength of the glenohumeral joint and scapula. Since the versatility of the shoulder is so large, if one of these exercises does not feel right, back off and consult your physician or physical therapist.

Shoulder Sequence Part I: Weeks 1 and 2

1. *Urdvha hastasana* (hands-in-the-air pose)

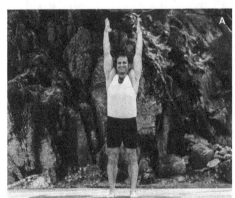 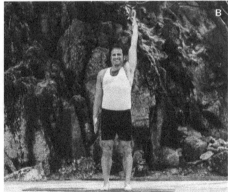

FIGURE 7.IA, B

a. Stand with your feet hip-width apart. Raise both arms directly overhead with the elbows straight and palms facing each other. Keep the arms equidistant from the ears. Pull the jawline backwards and keep the throat soft. Move the lower ribs backwards. Hold for 30 seconds.

b. Lift only one arm overhead and find its maximum pain-free range. Hold for 20 seconds. Repeat three times on each side.

156 APPLIED YOGA™ FOR MUSCULOSKELETAL PAIN

2. Arms at a T

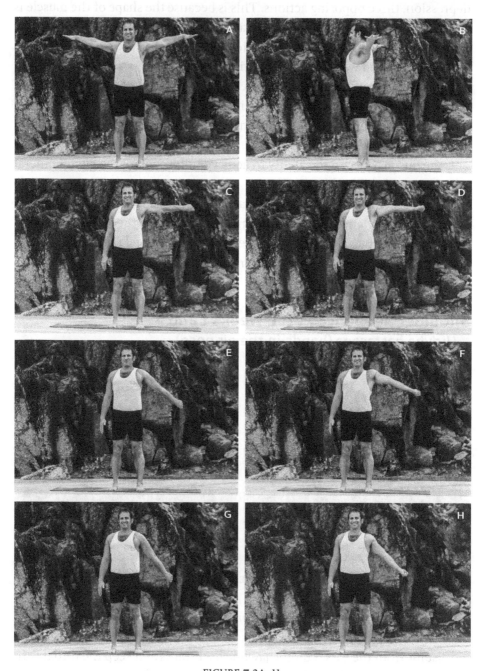

FIGURE 7.2A–H

a. Hold arms at 90° abduction. Lift the side ribs upwards and gently push the tailbone forward. Depress the shoulders away from the ears and straighten the elbows. Bring the arms backwards slightly so you can feel the shoulder blades moving towards each other (Figure 7.2a, b). Hold for 20–30 seconds. Bring arms back to your side.

b. Hold only one arm up and close the fist. Turn the shoulder in and out repeatedly to full pain-free range, exploring both internal and external rotation. Incrementally lower the arm as you continue to explore the rotation from different angles (Figure 7.2c–h).

3. *Gomukhasana* (cow face pose) lower arm isometric

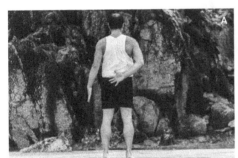 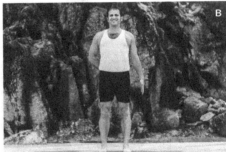

FIGURE 7.3A, B

a. Stand and place the back of the hand on top of the opposite buttock (if there is pain here, place hand on same-side buttock). Lift the chest and press the back of the hand into the buttock while rolling the outer shoulder backwards. Keep lifting the chest and slightly press the tailbone forward. Hold for 20–30 seconds.

b. Assume the same position and press the back of the hand into the back. Stabilize the hand on the back and drag the elbow out to the side to create traction inside the glenohumeral joint. Hold for 20–30 seconds.

Repeat on each side.

4. Pectoralis minor stretch on wall or floor

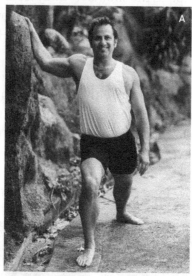

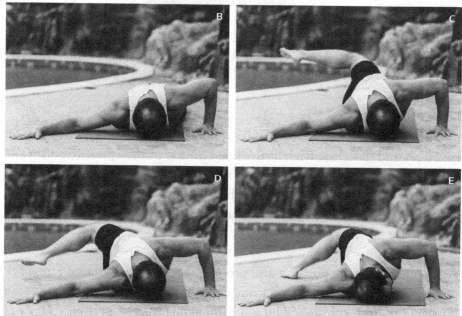

FIGURE 7.4A–E

a. Stand with the side of your body facing a wall. Bring the arm behind you at a 75° angle and place the palm on the wall. Step the leg nearest to the wall forward and slightly bend the front knee (Figure 7.4a). Hold for 15–20 seconds while breathing. Repeat two times on each side.

- **Variation on the floor:** Lie face down with the arm you want to stretch at your side and elbow bent to around 75°. Your other hand is near your shoulder, palm face down. Lift the opposite leg to your stretched arm and bring it across your body to your level of comfort (either flat on the ground or hovering in the air) (Figure 7.4b–e). Hold the stretch for 20–30 seconds. Repeat two times on each side.

5. *Bhujangasana* (cobra pose) lift-offs

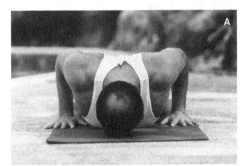
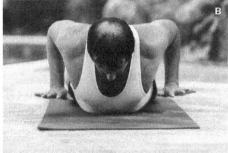

FIGURE 7.5A, B

a. Lie face down and place the palms by your chest, a little lower than the shoulders. Lift the head and chest, then lift the hands off the ground. Hold for five seconds. Repeat 5–8 times.

6. Prone external rotation with blocks

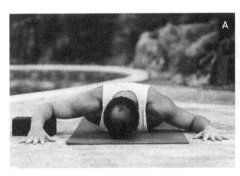
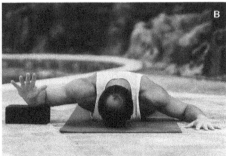

FIGURE 7.6A–B

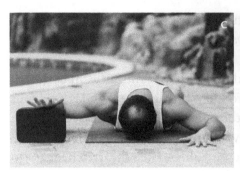 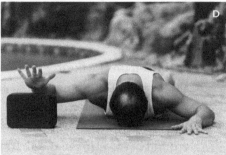

FIGURE 7.6C-D

a. Lie face down with one arm at 90°. Place a block under the tip of the elbow with the hand resting on the floor. Lift the forearm and hand as high as they can go while keeping the hand open and the wrist neutral. Repeat 3–5 times. At the top of each movement, pause and see if you can externally rotate the shoulder a little more. Repeat three times on each side.

- For a greater challenge, you can place a block under your wrist to passively position your shoulder in external rotation before activating it.

- For an even greater challenge, use a PNF contract-relax antagonist contract (CRAC) to increase the external rotator engagement. To do this, press downwards into the block at around 50 percent of your maximum force for 20 seconds. Immediately after, engage the external rotators and lift the wrist off the block to its maximum range. Hold for 10–20 seconds. Repeat at least twice.

7. *Savasana* (corpse pose)

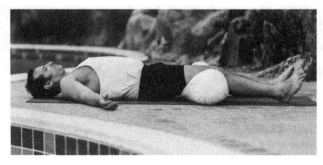

FIGURE 7.7

a. Lie on your back with a bolster under your knees. Stay for 3–10 minutes.

Shoulder Sequence Part II: Weeks 3 and 4

1. Pectoralis minor stretch on wall

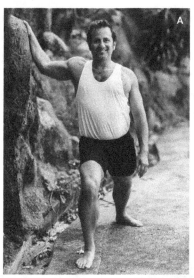

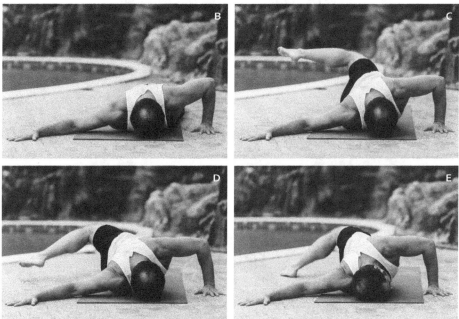

FIGURE 7.8A–E

a. Stand with the side of your body facing a wall. Bring the arm behind you at a 75° angle and place the palm on the wall. Step the leg nearest to the wall forward and slightly bend the front knee (Figure 7.8a). Hold for 15–20 seconds while breathing. Repeat two times on each side.

- **Variation on the floor:** Lie face down with the arm you want to stretch at your side and elbow bent to around 75°. Your other hand is near your shoulder, palm face down. Lift the opposite leg to your stretched arm and bring it across your body to your level of comfort (either flat on the ground or hovering in the air) (Figure 7.8b–e). Hold the stretch for 20–30 seconds. Repeat two times on each side.

2. Rhomboid and middle trapezius lift-offs

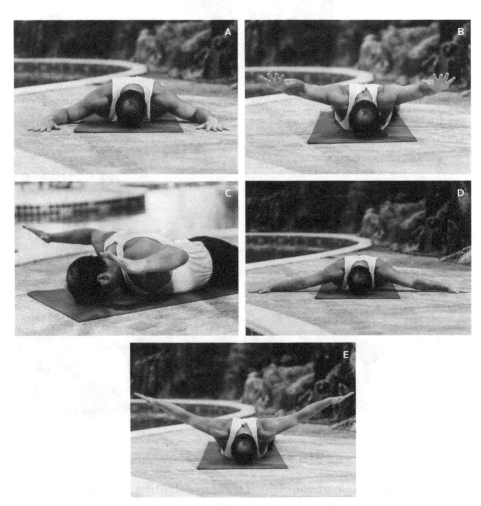

FIGURE 7.9A–E

a. **Rhomboid lift-offs:** Lie face down with your forehead on the floor and chin tucked (this prevents the back of your neck from gripping and strengthens the deep neck flexors). Bend the elbows to 90° and place the palms on the floor. Lift the bent arms upwards as high as you can go (Figure 7.9a–c). Hold for 15–20 seconds. As you hold, continually check to see if you can lift a little higher. Repeat 2–3 times.

b. **Middle trapezius lift-offs:** Lie face down with your forehead on the floor and chin tucked. Abduct the arms to 90° with elbows straight and lift them as high as you can go while retracting both scapulae (Figure 7.9d, e). Hold for 15–20 seconds. As you hold, continually check to see if you can lift a little higher. Repeat 2–3 times.

- **Note:** The arms will want to adduct and move closer to the hips. Don't let them. Keep them at 90° for maximal middle trapezius activation.

3. Prone wall angel

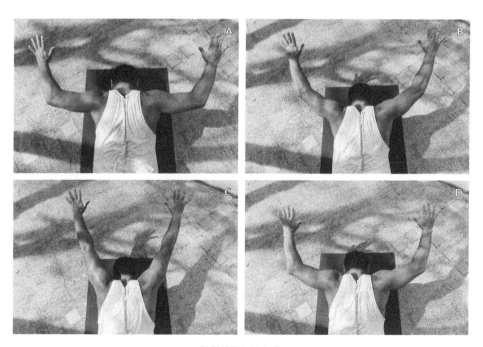

FIGURE 7.10A–D

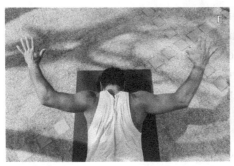
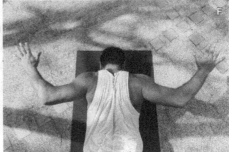

FIGURE 7.10E–F

a. Lie face down with your arms at 90° and forehead on the ground. Tuck the chin. Lift the arms as high as you can, bringing the shoulder blades together. Straighten the arms overhead, maintaining the height throughout the action. Then bend the elbows back and bring them towards the ribs to engage the latissimus dorsi muscles. Repeat 3–5 times.

4. Swimmers

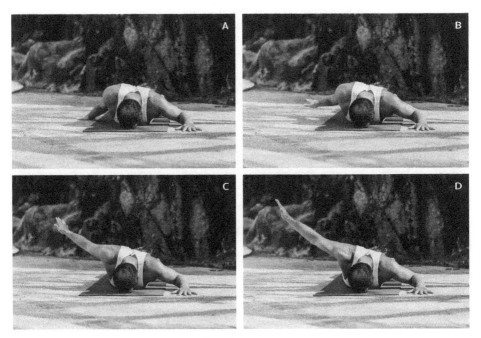

FIGURE 7.11A–D

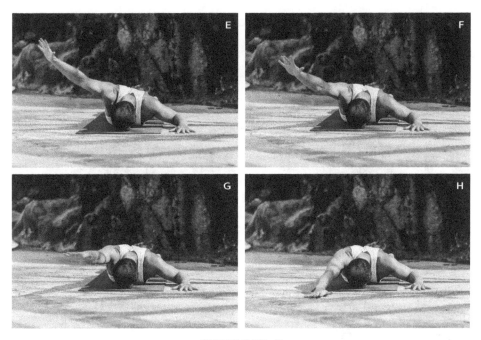

FIGURE 7.11E–H

a. Lie face down with one arm bent at 90° overhead and the other at your side. Lift the arm at your side as high as you can and bring it overhead as if you were swimming. Keep the arm as high as possible throughout the entire motion so you can train the shoulder's full range. Repeat 3–5 times on each side.

- **Tip:** At the points where you feel the arm drop, pause and lift it more. This will create more strength.

5. Prone external rotation with blocks

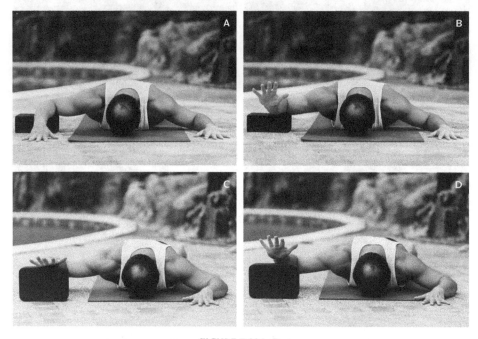

FIGURE 7.12A–D

a. Lie face down with one arm at 90°. Place a block under the tip of the elbow with the hand resting on the floor. Lift the forearm and hand as high as they can go while keeping the hand open and the wrist neutral. Repeat 3–5 times. At the top of each movement, pause and see if you can externally rotate the shoulder a little more. Repeat three times on each side.

- For a greater challenge, you can place a block under your wrist to passively position your shoulder in external rotation before activating it.

- For an even greater challenge, use a PNF contract-relax antagonist contract (CRAC) to increase the external rotator engagement. To do this, press downwards into the block at around 50 percent of your maximum force for 20 seconds. Immediately after, engage the external rotators and lift the wrist off the block to its maximum range. Hold for 10–20 seconds. Repeat at least twice.

6. Forearm plank walks

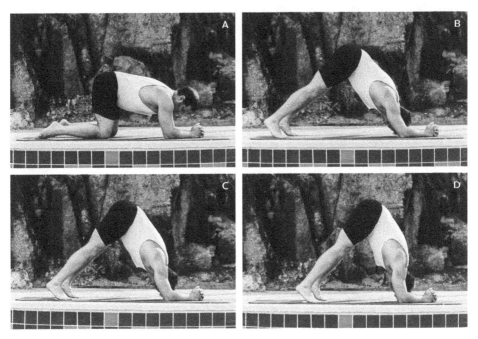

FIGURE 7.13A–D

a. Assume a triangular-shaped forearm plank by interlacing the fingers and placing the forearms on the ground with the legs straight behind you and buttocks high in the air. Walk the feet towards the hands about six inches and pause. Take three breaths. Repeat this two more times until you cannot walk in any further. Walk backwards and rest. Repeat two times.

7. *Savasana* (corpse pose)

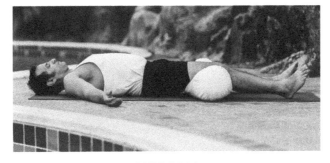

FIGURE 7.14

a. Lie on your back with a bolster under your knees. Stay for 3–10 minutes.

CHAPTER 8

Anatomy of the Neck

The neck is the most flexible part of the spine. There are seven cervical vertebrae that form a natural inward curve, called lordosis. This is the same direction of curve as the lower back. The upper two cervical vertebrae are smaller and more mobile than the five below them. This is a design that allows those five lower vertebrae, C3–C7, to handle heavier loads from the head and neck. The head itself weighs around 8–12 pounds and in total there are nearly 30 muscles that help move and stabilize the neck. The primary motions of the neck are flexion, extension, rotation, and side bending.

C1–C2, the uppermost cervical vertebrae, are considered atypical because they have different shapes compared to the rest of the spine. C1, known as the atlas, has no spinous process and a ring around it that connects to the occipital bone of the skull above it. This junction forms the atlanto-occipital joint. Much of the neck's flexion and extension occurs here.

The C2 vertebra, called the axis, has a large bony protrusion known as the dens. The dens fits into the ring-shaped atlas above it, forming the atlanto-axial joint. This is the spine's most mobile joint and as much as 60 percent of the head's rotational motion occurs here.

C3–C6 are considered normal vertebrae because they share similar features with the rest of the spine, such as facet joints and articular cartilage, which allow for smooth movement. They are primarily involved in lateral flexion or side bending of the neck.

C7, the end of the cervical portion of the spine, is the largest of the cervical vertebrae and has a longer spinous process than the others. If you touch the lower portion of the back of your neck and feel the vertebra that protrudes the most, you are most likely touching the C7 vertebrae. Its elongated size allows more muscles to attach to it than any other cervical vertebra.

There are eight pairs of cervical nerves. Each one is supplied by two nerve roots. The anterior root carries motor signals from the brain out to the body.

The posterior root carries sensory signals from the body back to the brain. The head, neck, shoulder, elbow, wrist, and hand are all innervated by the cervical nerves.

The phrenic nerve, briefly spoken about in Chapter 3, originates from the C3–C5 nerve roots. It sends motor signals to the diaphragm so that we can breathe and receives sensory information in return. This is where the phrase "C3–5 keeps the diaphragm alive" comes from. There is a right and left phrenic nerve. The right phrenic nerve runs superficial to the anterior scalene—an accessory muscle of respiration—and terminates in the diaphragmatic opening at T8. The left phrenic nerve terminates at the central tendon of the diaphragm. Damage to this nerve can significantly affect our breathing patterns.

One of the more common dysfunctions of the neck is something called forward head posture (FHP). FHP is a condition where the lower cervical spine moves into flexion while the upper cervical spine moves into hyperextension. This causes the center of gravity in the head to be forward from where it's supposed to be and not centered directly over the vertebral bodies. It is proposed that this makes the head feel as though it weighs as much as three times more than it actually does.

FHP has been shown to correlate with respiratory muscle weakness.[1] The amount of oxygen intake and carbon dioxide expulsion decreases with FHP.[2] Nasal breathing patterns often transform into mouth breathing, and two accessory muscles of respiration, the scalenes and sternocleidomastoid, show higher than normal activity.[3] If this weren't enough, a decrease in range of motion and neck flexor strength, and an increase in neck muscle fatigue are commonly shown.[4]

FHP has increased over the last 20 years due to smartphones, long hours at the desk, and long commutes in the car. Poor posture, however, has been part of the human condition since our existence. Gravity is pulling us down, and emotional factors such as depression play a key role in how we hold ourselves. Addressing your posture through the sequences in this book can be a pivotal factor in restoring your musculoskeletal health and freeing your neck from discomfort.

Neck pain in general is one of the most common musculoskeletal disorders, second only to low back pain.[5] It's estimated that around 30–50 percent of people will complain of neck pain each year. What happens in the neck, however, is rarely the fault of the neck alone. Our thoracic spine's posture, the position of the scapula, and the mobility of the glenohumeral joint all play significant roles in how our necks feel and move.

One particular shoulder muscle, the pectoralis minor, is commonly implicated in neck pain. The pectoralis minor originates on the 3rd–5th ribs and attaches on the coracoid process. Its primary function is to stabilize and protract the scapula. An overly taut pectoralis minor is the primary cause of scapular dyskinesis, or an alteration of the normal resting position of the scapula. This affects the neck greatly and can be a factor in the arising of another common condition, called upper crossed syndrome (UCS).

UCS, similar to FHP, will present as a hunching of the thoracic spine and rounding of the shoulders. The pectoralis minor/major, levator, and upper trapezius will be tight while the deep neck flexors, rhomboids, and lower trapezius will be weak.

Addressing only the muscular components without creating proper alignment of the scapula and thoracic spine will provide only limited results. Similarly, when the glenohumeral joint of the shoulder lacks either internal or external rotation, it will affect the function of everything around it and can be a key factor in creating neck pain.

You will find two unique approaches to neck pain in this chapter. The first is the creation of thoracic and cervical flexion. This is counterintuitive to what is commonly taught in yoga classes and physical therapy exercises. Much of yoga is centered around creating extension of the thoracic spine to counteract our poor posture. This is vitally important and a boon granted upon us by the yoga system. But the focus on creating thoracic extension has also created a demonization of thoracic and cervical flexion. This is where we have failed as movement experts.

Since the atlanto-occipital (OA) joint is commonly stuck in extension, causing the suboccipitals and other cervical muscles to be tight, it makes sense to teach it how to flex properly. There is no amount of massage or chiropractic adjustment that will hold unless the movement capacity of the joint is changed. Focusing solely on increasing one range of motion and not the other deprives our body of its full ranges. When this happens, it affects our musculoskeletal system and our psyche. If we are always trying to open and refusing to consciously close, a movement imbalance is created.

The spine is healthiest when it is fluid. This means that all 24 vertebrae move harmoniously with one another. Making our thoracic and cervical spines fully round with a protracted scapula provides a stretch to the connecting musculature. The freedom that comes to the chronically stuck OA joint reveals other segments of the spine that are immobile. In this way, we allow flexion of the OA to be the teacher and inform the other vertebrae of their direct limitations. These other vertebrae then reinform the OA in a symbiotic healing relationship.

Second is the practice of the neck circles. Neck circles were all the rage in the 1980s and their intention was good—to create full range of motion in the cervical spine. But it was found that they were actually causing people more pain and they quickly became a taboo movement. The pain was a result of a spinal compression taking place in the lower cervical vertebrae. This compression, as you may have guessed, was strongly influenced by forward head posture, upper crossed syndrome, and thoracic kyphosis. When the cervical vertebrae are already mispositioned anteriorly and the thoracic spine hunched posteriorly, doing a neck circle is a breeding ground for more dysfunction.

There are two healthy ways to do a neck circle. The first is to perform them with limited range and zero pain as a way to send a signal to the brain that the neck can move pain-free. This is especially beneficial after a minor neck injury—such as after sleeping poorly or when you get one of those stingers—to prevent catastrophizing or kinesiophobia. Remember, RICE is not the answer. We want to teach ourselves how to move pain-free.

The other way to perform a neck circle is to do so with different positioning of the thoracic spine, scapula, and glenohumeral joint. It is commonly found that a previously painful neck circle becomes pain-free with a new alignment of one of these areas. This shows us that the pain we are experiencing in the neck has its root cause somewhere else. We will explore the relationship of these three areas to all the ranges of motion of the neck.

Of note is that you may find particular stretches from the shoulder section of this book to be especially helpful for the neck. This is where your intelligence and knowledge of your unique body come into play. Whatever you find that works, please feel free to incorporate and practice it regularly. There is no one who knows your body better than you.

My recommendation with this sequence is to practice it and find specifically what works for you. Some will need scapular retraction, others thoracic extension, and some will need more glenohumeral rotation. Once you find what alleviates your pain, repeat the sequence four times a week for maximal results.

Neck Sequence
1. Neck range-of-motion assessment

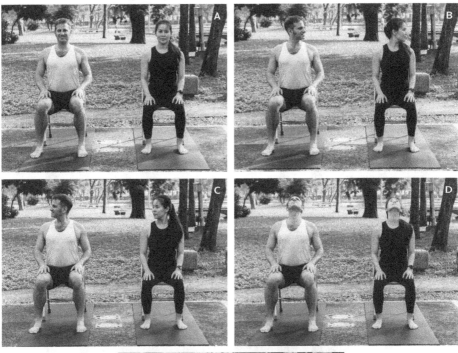

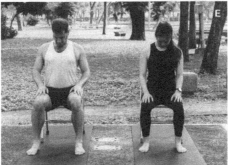

FIGURE 8.1A–E

a. Sit on a chair and lift your chest (Figure 8.1a). Close your eyes and take your mind to the top of your head. Turn your head slowly left and right to assess your cervical rotation (Figure 8.1b, c). Do not tuck your chin or rotate your ribs. Then tilt your head upwards and downwards to assess flexion and extension (Figure 8.1d, e).

– You will often notice one side of the rotation being more difficult than the other or one of the flexion/extension ranges being limited. This is going to be your range of motion to work on and correct. We are now going to assess if repositioning the scapula, glenohumeral joint, or thoracic spine positively affects your neck's range of motion. If it does, you will continue to practice the exact exercise that helps.

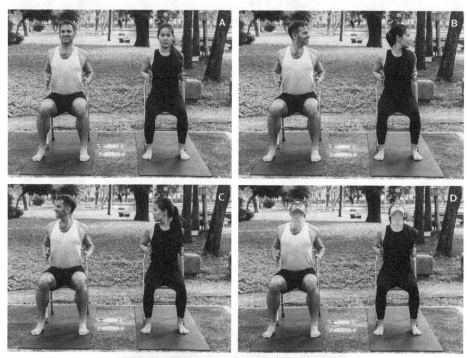

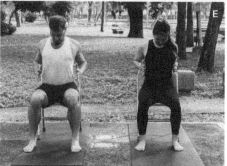

FIGURE 8.2A–E

b. Bend the elbows and retract the scapula. Keep the elbows close to your ribs and the palms facing towards each other (Figure 8.2a). Turn the head left and right, assessing if this scapula-retracted position helps cervical rotation (Figure 8.2b, c). Then tilt it upwards and downwards to assess extension and flexion (Figure 8.2d, e).

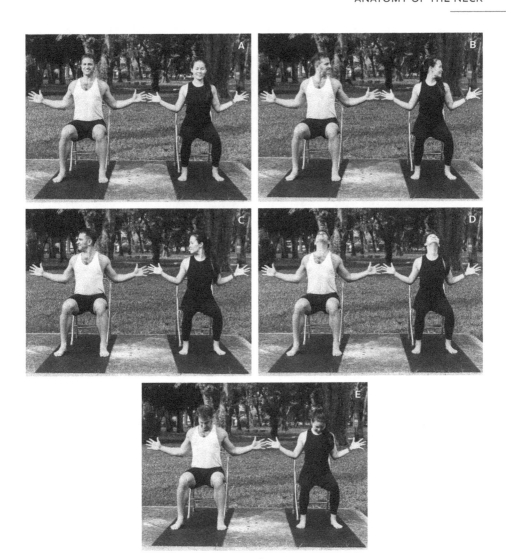

FIGURE 8.3A–E

c. Bend your elbows and put them at your sides. Externally rotate the shoulders by taking the forearms backwards. Assess the external rotation of each shoulder to see if one is more limited than the other. If it is, put extra attention on that joint to create more external rotation. Turn the head left, right, up, and down to assess rotation.

176 APPLIED YOGA™ FOR MUSCULOSKELETAL PAIN

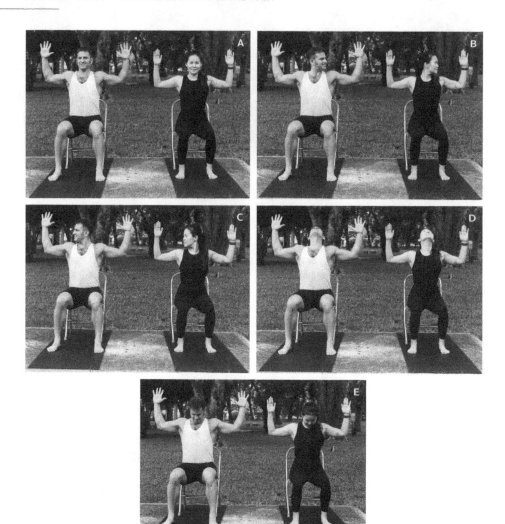

FIGURE 8.4A–E

d. Put your arms into 90° angles. Look at each arm to make sure they are equal. Turn your head left, right, up, and down.

- **Note:** If this position has helped, it often means that the pectoralis minor is also tight and the shoulder is rounded slightly forward. Adding the pectoralis minor stretch from the shoulder section may help.

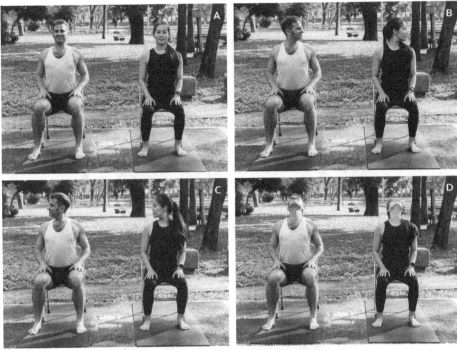
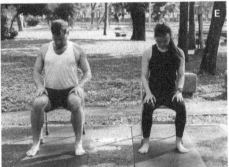

FIGURE 8.5A–E

e. Place your hands on your upper thighs and lift your chest as much as you can to create thoracic extension. Turn your head left, right, up, and down.

f. Whichever range of motion was limited for you and whichever exercise helped it the most, repeat that until the range of motion has shifted in the moment. Then continue that exercise four times a week until it has resolved and a new range of motion is established.

2. Neck circles

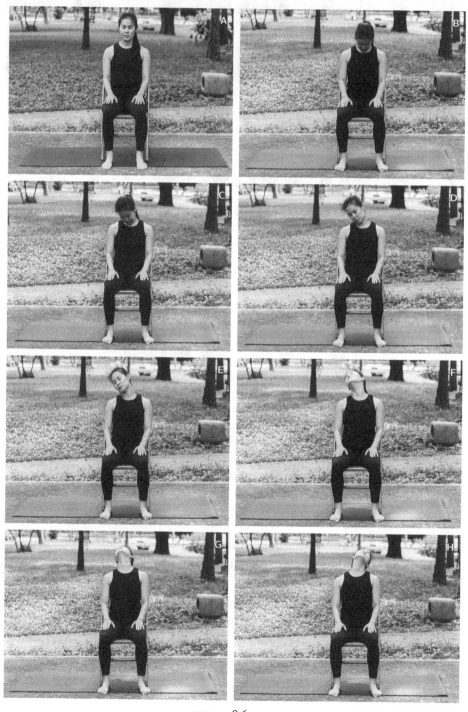

FIGURE 8.6A–H

ANATOMY OF THE NECK 179

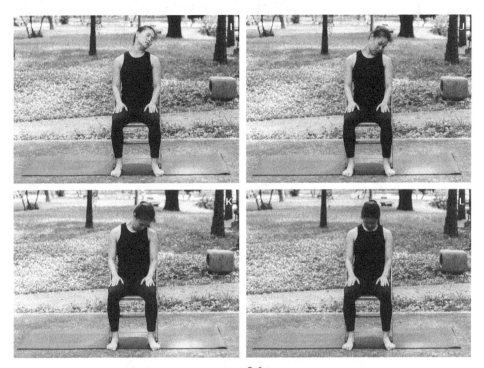

FIGURE 8.61-L

a. Sit on a chair and lift your chest. Take your head downwards (keeping your chest lifted) and trace the clavicle with your chin as you begin a neck circle. Do not rotate the ribs. Perform one circle in each direction as an assessment only. Make a note of any pain points.

- Pain in the back of the neck when doing a neck circle is often because of joint compression so we are using this initial circle solely for assessment and then to see if we can make the appropriate changes based on scapular, glenohumeral, or thoracic vertebral shifts.

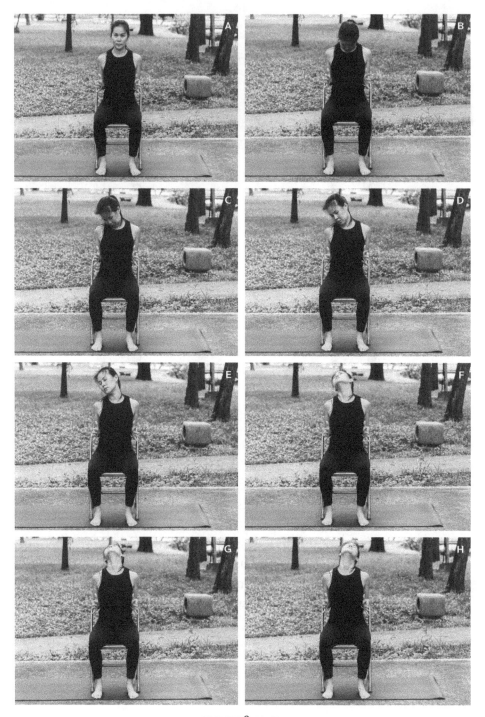

FIGURE 8.7A–H

ANATOMY OF THE NECK 181

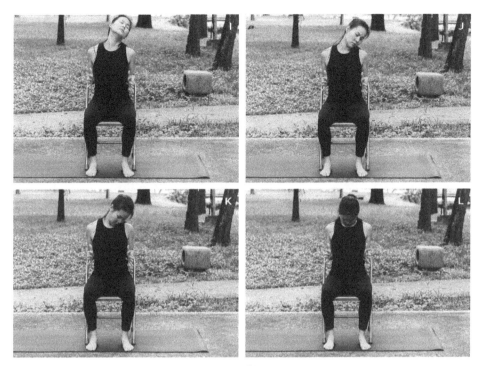

FIGURE 8.71–L

b. Bend the elbows and retract the scapula. Keep the elbows close to your ribs and the palms facing each other. Perform a neck circle and see if the pain has dissipated. If it has, continue with this motion. If it has not, you may stop and proceed to the next action.

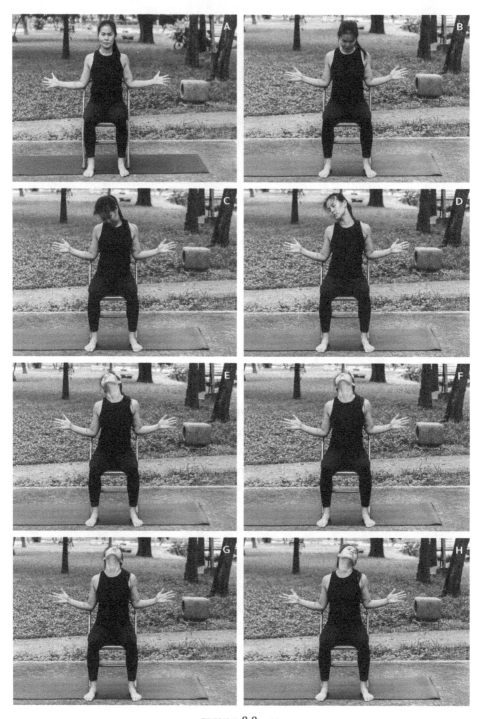

FIGURE 8.8A–H

ANATOMY OF THE NECK 183

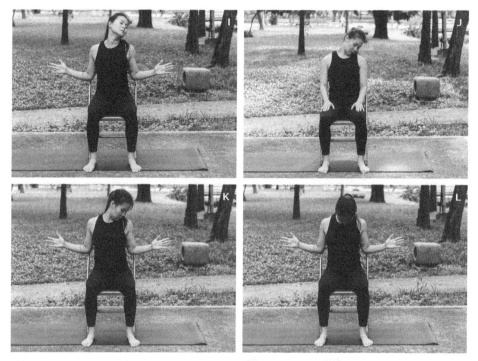

FIGURE 8.81-L

c. Bend your elbows and put them at your sides. Externally rotate the shoulders by taking the forearms backwards. Make each arm equal. Perform a neck circle and see if the pain has dissipated. If it has, continue with this motion. If it has not, you may stop and proceed to the next action.

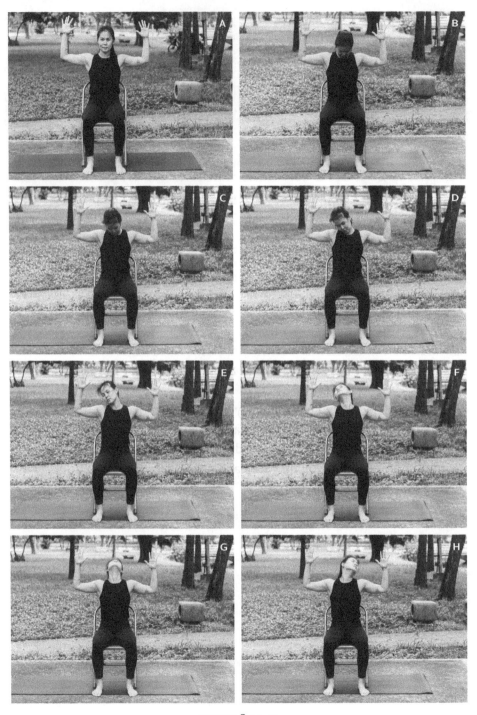

FIGURE 8.9A–H

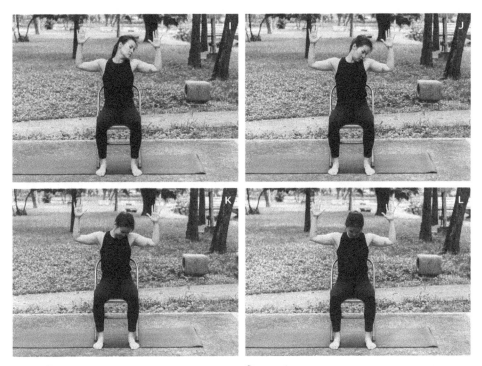

FIGURE 8.91–L

d. Put your arms into 90° angles and make them equal. Perform a neck circle and see if the pain has dissipated. If it has, continue with this motion. If it has not, you may stop and proceed to the next action.

186 APPLIED YOGA™ FOR MUSCULOSKELETAL PAIN

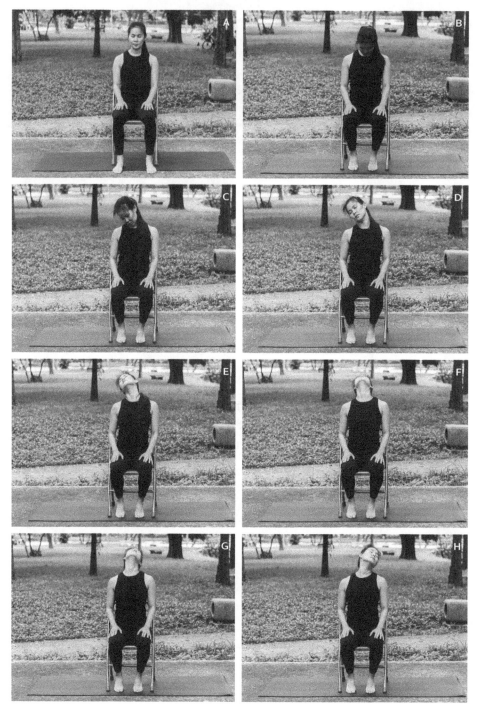

FIGURE 8.10A–H

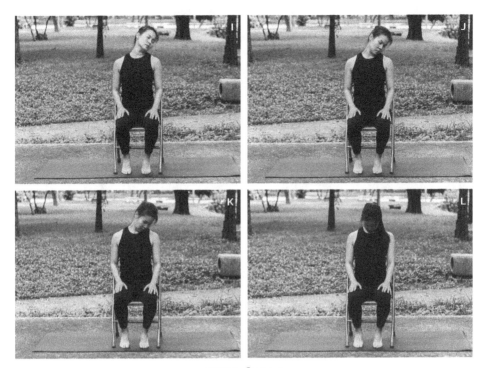

FIGURE 8.10A-1

e. Place your hands on your upper thighs and lift your chest as much as you can to create thoracic extension. Perform a neck circle to see if the pain has dissipated.

f. Whichever action allows your neck to feel the freest when doing a neck circle is the one to continue. If none of them helped, you can do a minimal range circle and avoid any pain points. This sends a signal to your brain that your neck can move pain-free. Repeat whatever works, doing three circles in each direction four times a week.

3. Cervical and thoracic rounding

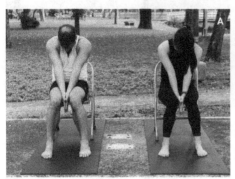
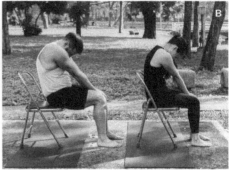

FIGURE 8.11A, B

a. Sit on a chair and place your hands together, in between your knees. Squeeze the hands together with your knees, round your head, and round your upper back. This will stretch the upper back and neck muscles. Use the knees to pin the hands and create leverage for you to push your upper back backwards. Hold for 10–15 seconds.

b. Release the hands and place them on the back of the head (Figure 8.12). Gently press the head downwards to stretch the muscles on the back of your neck. Hold for 10–15 seconds.

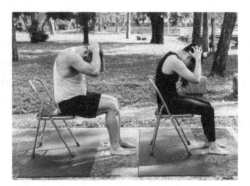

FIGURE 8.12

c. After performing both of these, sit tall and lift the chest.

4. Rhomboid stretch

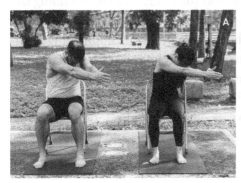
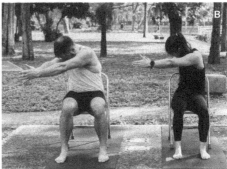

FIGURE 8.13A, B

a. Sit on a chair, round the upper back and neck, and place the arms in front of you with the palms together. Twist to one side, reaching both arms in the same direction to receive a stretch in the rhomboid. Hold for 10–15 seconds. Repeat two times on each side.

5. Cervical traction from *uttanasana* (standing forward fold)

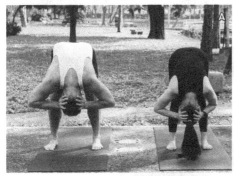
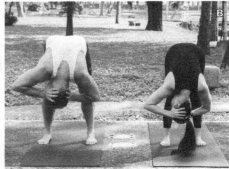
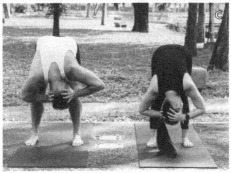

FIGURE 8.14A–C

a. Stand with your feet hip-width apart and bend your knees as much as necessary to comfortably rest your hands on the floor. (We are not doing this for a hamstring stretch.) Grab hold of your head with each hand just above the ear. The ear drum should not be covered and your middle fingers are facing towards each other, just beneath the occiput. (To find the occiput, place your hand on the back of your head and find the bony protuberance. That's the occiput.) Pull your head downwards and tuck the chin to traction the cervical spine. Hold for only 5–10 seconds but do this repeatedly before coming up. Turn the head slightly to the right or left and repeat the same action there.

6. Cervical rotations supine

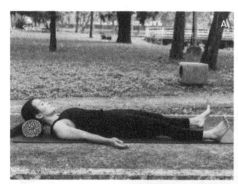
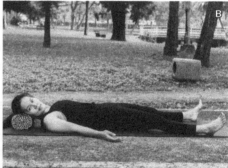
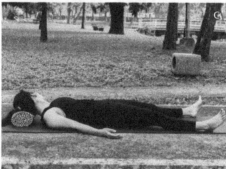

FIGURE 8.15A–C

a. Lie down with your occiput on a rolled blanket. Slowly turn your head to the left and right while keeping your occiput on the blanket at all times. You will find that your occiput wants to move off the blanket. Keeping it on ensures you're rotating from the atlanto-axial joint and not compressing other vertebrae.

Repeat three times on each side. If one side is limited, repeat that side until the desired range is found.

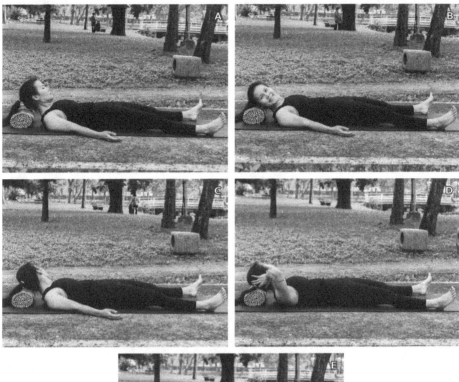

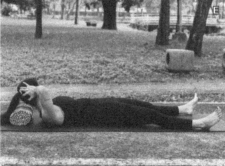

FIGURE 8.16A–E

b. **Advanced:** Lift your head off the blanket and turn it to the right and left (Figure 8.16a–c). If you feel one direction is limited, stay there and see if you can rotate more.

When you find the direction that's limited, pause and place your hand on the back of your head (Figure 8.16d, e). Flex and extend your neck a few times while providing resistance with your hand. Then see if your range of motion has changed.

7. Chin tucks while supine

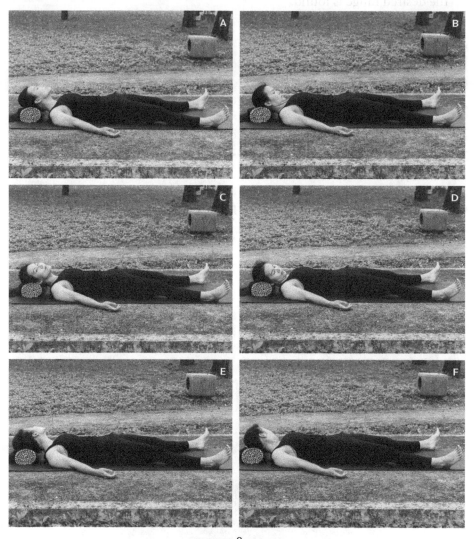

FIGURE 8.17A–F

a. Roll a blanket and place it directly under the occiput (Figure 8.17a, b). Press the back of the head into the blanket while tucking the chin. Repeat 5–8 times. On the final repetition, hold the position for five seconds.

b. Turn the head 45° to the side and press it backwards into the blanket while tucking the chin (Figure 8.17c–f). Repeat 5–8 times. On the final repetition, hold the position for five seconds.

Repeat on the other side.

8. Ace bandage *setu bhandasana* (bridge pose)

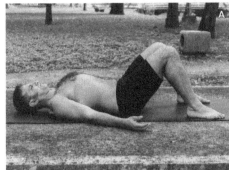
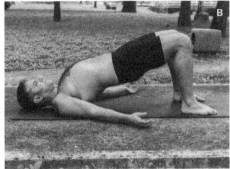
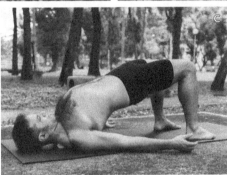

FIGURE 8.18A–C

a. Lie on the floor with an ace bandage placed horizontally underneath C7. (To locate C7, place your hand on the base of your neck. There is a vertebra that is more prominent that the others. That is C7.) Bend both knees and lift your hips into *setu bhandasana*. Pressurize the C7 vertebra into the ace bandage. Hold 20–30 seconds.

- **Note:** You may also find it helpful to position the bandage anywhere from T1–T3, as well.

9. Backbend with the blanket/blocks

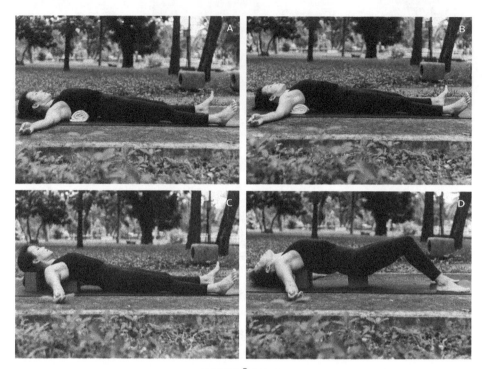

FIGURE 8.19A–D

a. Backbend with the blanket: Roll a blanket and place it horizontal to your spine (Figure 8.19a, b). Lie back, with the blanket around the T7–T8 vertebrae, your head on the ground and arms above the blanket. Rest here and breathe for 1–2 minutes. Move downwards slightly so the blanket is now around T4–T5. Stay here for 1–2 minutes. You may continue to place the blanket around any thoracic vertebrae that feel stuck and need mobilization.

b. For backbend with the blocks (Figure 8.19c–d), place two blocks on the ground, one at the lowest height and one at the second height (Figure 8.19c). Lie backwards so the lower block is connected to your thoracic region and the upper block is supporting your head. Stay for 1–3 minutes.

  - **Advanced:** Place one block at the second height and lie backwards on it around the level of T7–T8. Lift your hips and place a block at the lowest height under your buttocks. Take your arms out to the sides or over your head (Figure 8.18d). This is a very strong thoracic extension exercise. Stay as long as you are comfortable.

10. *Savasana* (corpse pose)

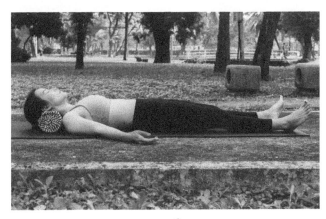

FIGURE 8.20

a. Roll a blanket and place it under your neck for *savasana*. Stay for 3–10 minutes.

10. Savasana (corpse pose).

CHAPTER 9

Bonus Section: Sacroiliac Joint and Glute Strength

The sacroiliac (SI) joint is the articulation of the sacrum with the part of our pelvis known as the ilium. It is the transition point between the spine, pelvis, and the lower body. Its role is to dissipate the distribution of force and act as a shock absorber between the lower body and the spine.

The SI joint is very small, ranging somewhere from 0.5 mm to 4 mm (0.02"–0.16") (in space). It is supported by the anterior, posterior, and interosseus sacroiliac ligaments as well as the sacrotuberous and sacrospinous ligaments. Motion of the joint is quite limited, and its ranges are debated, but includes around 3 degrees of flexion/extension, 1.5 degrees of rotation, and 0.8 degrees of lateral flexion.

The SI joint is commonly blamed for lower back pain but it is less involved than people may think. People will often say their SI joint hurts but then point to their lumbar vertebrae, not their sacral vertebrae, to show where their discomfort is. SI joint pain is commonly felt along the line of the sacrum with referral patterns into the legs. It can even mimic sciatica at times.

There are a variety of orthopedic tests to diagnose SIJD (sacroiliac joint dysfunction) but none that provide concrete evidence. The most effective technique for diagnosing SIJD is a local injection of anesthesia into the joint that results in a 75 percent decrease in pain. This is often repeated twice to fully confirm the findings.

Despite the difficulty in accurate assessment, one consistent attribute of SIJD is a combination of weak glutes and weak transversus abdominus.

The gluteus maximus has attachments on the sacrum that contribute to stabilizing the SI joint. Studies have shown that individuals with SIJD demonstrate inefficient gluteus maximus recruitment during weight-bearing activities.[1] Weakness of the gluteus maximus can thus be related to abnormal loading of the SI joint and cause pain. Glute activation, as little as 30 minutes twice a week for five weeks, has a significant impact on glute strength, and SI and lumbopelvic pain.[2]

The gluteus medius is a stabilizer of the hip and has attachments on the greater trochanter and ilium. It has a tendency to become short, weak, and tight. It is a complex muscle because even though it is tight, releasing it through soft tissue work or stretching only provides minimal, short-term relief. The common deficiency in neural drive to the gluteus medius, combined with the fact that stretching a weak muscle often makes it weaker, means the gluteus medius requires both release and activation to provide adequate stability and mobility to the hip.

When it is underactive and shortens, the ilium shifts upwards creating a minor mispositioning of the sacrum and compressing the SI joint. Lengthening and strengthening of the gluteus medius is thus paramount for healing SIJD.

Activation of the transversus abdominus has been shown to decrease laxity and stabilize the SI joint.[3] Thus, it should also be included in all SI joint sequences.

The following is a three-week sequence, as opposed to the four weeks of all previous sections. It is my suggestion that you do it 3–4 days a week to help strengthen the glutes and stabilize the SI joint. If you have true SI pain, there is a chance it will be relieved before the three weeks are done; if so, feel free to repeat only as needed. Anything from this section may also be added to the low back sequence because of the intimate relationship between the SI joint and lumbar spine.

Glute Sequence: Weeks 1–3
1. Turkish get up

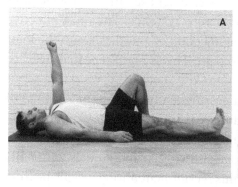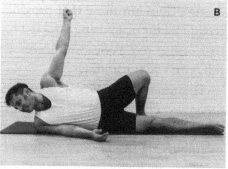

FIGURE 9.1A, B

a. Lie on your back and bend one knee. Lift the ipsilateral arm towards the ceiling. Press the foot of the bent knee downwards into the ground and lift the hip and head up while turning the body to the opposite side. Do not let the knee follow this direction, however, and keep it perpendicular to the floor. Reach the arm towards the ceiling. Repeat five times. Do one set on each side.

2. Side-lying leg lifts

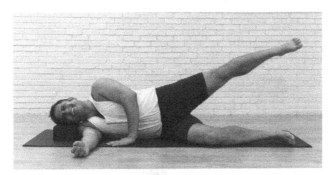

FIGURE 9.2

a. Lie on your side and make your body straight. Bend the bottom knee. Lift the top leg to its maximum height without rolling the hip backwards or externally rotating the thigh.

- Lengthen your hip from the top of the ilium to the greater trochanter. This is a very subtle action. I am asking you to visualize and lengthen the gluteus medius and tensor fascia latae. It is easy to lengthen the lower back here and get a stretch in the quadratus lumborum. That is not what we're doing. We are getting way more specific than that. Hold this for 30–60 seconds and repeat two times.

3. Mini bridge pose

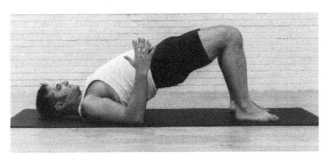

FIGURE 9.3

a. Lie on your back and bend both knees. Press the affected side's foot into the floor and lift the hips only a couple inches off the ground. Do not press down with the other foot. Posteriorly tuck your pelvis to lengthen your lower back. Progressively engage the gluteus maximus by increasing the strength of foot pressure into the floor. Relax the toes and press the big toe mound down. Hold for 30–60 seconds with the focus on unilateral glute engagement. Repeat 2–3 times.

4. Donkey kicks

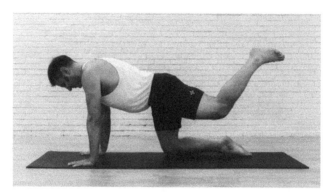

FIGURE 9.4

a. From the quadruped position, put a slight grip into the lower abdomen and lift one leg into the air while keeping the knee bent. Maintain the opposite hip directly over the knee. Slightly externally rotate the lifted leg. *Do not overarch or twist the lower back.* Lift the leg until maximum range and glute contraction is felt. Hold for 15–20 seconds. Repeat two times on each side.

5. Figure 4

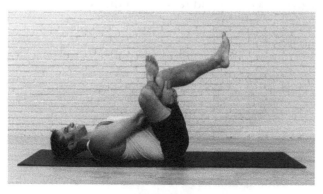

FIGURE 9.5

a. Lie on your back with both knees bent. Cross one ankle over the top of the opposite knee. Bring the legs into the air and grab behind the knee. Keep that knee around a 110° angle. This aids in the stretch. Hold for 20–30 seconds.

Repeat on the other side.

- **Tip:** Slightly rock your pelvis away from the crossed leg (if your right hip is being stretched, rock gently to the left). This will increase the stretch in the hip.

6. *Virabhadrasana II* (warrior II)

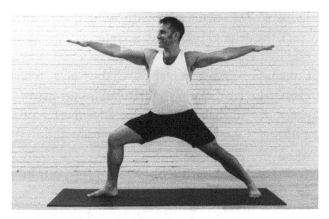

FIGURE 9.6

a. Separate the feet 3½–4½ feet apart. Align the front heel with the back arch. Bend the knee until you make a right angle with your hip, knee, and foot. Press the front heel down to increase the engagement of the gluteus maximus. Hold for 20–30 seconds. Repeat two times on each side.

7. Plank pose

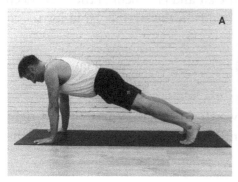 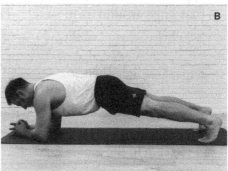

FIGURE 9.7

a. Straight arm plank: Take plank pose with straight arms and straight legs. Posteriorly tuck the pelvis. Hold for 20 seconds.

b. Forearm plank: Assume forearm plank with the fingers interlaced and the elbows spread. On each exhalation, pull the belly button towards the spine. This will engage the transversus abdominus. Do five breaths. Repeat each pose three times.

8. *Savasana* (corpse pose) with a bolster under your knees

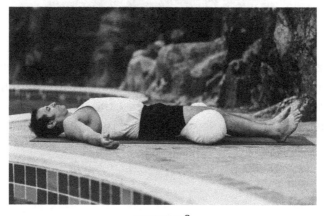

FIGURE 9.8

a. Lie on your back with a bolster under your knees. Stay for 3–10 minutes.

Endnotes

Chapter 1

1 Penman, S., Cohen, S., Stevens, P., and Jackson, S. (2012) Yoga in Australia: Results of a national survey. *International Journal of Yoga 5*, 2, 92–101. www.ncbi.nlm.nih.gov/pmc/articles/PMC3410203

2 Penman, S., Cohen, S., Stevens, P., and Jackson, S. (2012) Yoga in Australia: Results of a national survey. *International Journal of Yoga 5*, 2, 92–101. www.ncbi.nlm.nih.gov/pmc/articles/PMC3410203

3 Times of India (2015) World's oldest yoga centre still going strong. https://timesofindia.indiatimes.com/city/mumbai/Worlds-oldest-yoga-centre-still-going-strong/articleshow/36904643.cms

4 Mangalore Today News Network (2009) Yoga guru Pattabhi Jois accused of sexual assault in new photos. www.mangaloretoday.com/titbits/Yoga-guru-Pattabhi-Jois-accused-of-sexual-assault-in-new-photos.html

5 Godwin, R. (2017) "He said he could do what he wanted": The scandal that rocked Bikram yoga. *The Guardian*, February 18. www.theguardian.com/lifeandstyle/2017/feb/18/bikram-hot-yoga-scandal-choudhury-what-he-wanted

   Schettler, R.M. (2023) He faced allegations of sexual assault and rape from students for years. Now Bikram Choudhury is "back" teaching in Canada. Outside, February 9. www.yogajournal.com/lifestyle/bikram-choudhury-teaching-yoga

6 Mikkonen, J., Pederson, P., and McCarthy, P.W. (2008) A survey of musculoskeletal injury among Ashtanga Vinyasa Yoga practitioners. *International Journal of Yoga Therapy 18*, 1, 59–64. https://doi.org/10.17761/ijyt.18.1.l0748p25k2558v77

7 Hirsch, R. (2017) The opioid epidemic: It's time to place blame where it belongs. *Missouri Medicine 114*, 2, 82–83. www.ncbi.nlm.nih.gov/pmc/articles/PMC6140023

   Mann, B. and Bebinger, M. (2022) Purdue Pharma, Sacklers reach $6 billion deal with state attorneys general. NPR, March 3. www.npr.org/2022/03/03/1084163626/purdue-sacklers-oxycontin-settlement

8 Tabish, S.A. (2008) Complementary and alternative healthcare: Is it evidence-based? *International Journal of Health Sciences 2*, 1, v–ix. www.ncbi.nlm.nih.gov/pmc/articles/PMC3068720

9 Beazley, D., Patel, S., Davis, B., Vinson, S., and Bolgla, L. (2017) Trunk and hip muscle activation during yoga poses: Implications for physical therapy practice. *Complementary Therapies in Clinical Practice 29*, 130-135. https://doi.org/10.1016/j.ctcp.2017.09.009

10 Williams, K., Abildso, C., Steinberg, L., Doyle, E. *et al.* (2009) Evaluation of the effectiveness and efficacy of Iyengar yoga therapy on chronic low back pain. *Spine 34*, 19, 2066-2076. https://doi.org/10.1097/brs.0b013e3181b315cc

11 Sherman, K., Cherkin, D.C., Erro, J., Miglioretti, D.L., and Deyo, R.A. (2005) Comparing yoga, exercise, and a self-care book for chronic low back pain: A randomized, controlled trial. *Annals of Internal Medicine 143*, 12, 849-856. https://doi.org/10.7326/0003-4819-143-12-200512200-00003

12 Ebnezar, J., Nagarathna, R., Yogitha, B., and Nagendra, H.R. (2012) Effects of an integrated approach of hatha yoga therapy on functional disability, pain, and flexibility in osteoarthritis of the knee joint: A randomized controlled study. *Journal of Alternative and Complementary Medicine 18*, 5, 463-472. https://doi.org/10.1089/acm.2010.0320

13 Garfinkel, M.S., Singhal, A., Katz, W.A., Allan, D.A., Reshetar, R., and Schumacher, H.R., Jr. (1998) Yoga-based intervention for carpal tunnel syndrome: A randomized trial. *JAMA 280*, 18, 1601-1603. https://doi.org/10.1001/jama.280.18.1601

14 Carson, J.W., Carson, K.M., Jones, K.D., Bennett, R.M., Wright, C.L., and Mist, S.D. (2010) A pilot randomized controlled trial of the Yoga of Awareness program in the management of fibromyalgia. *Pain 151*, 2, 530-539. https://doi.org/10.1016%2Fj.pain.2010.08.020

15 Groessl, E.J., Liu, L., Chang, D.G., Wetherell, J.L. *et al.* (2017) Yoga for military veterans with chronic low back pain: A randomized clinical trial. *American Journal of Preventive Medicine 53*, 5, 599-608. https://doi.org/10.1016/j.amepre.2017.05.019

16 McCaffrey, R., Frock, T.L., and Garguilo, H. (2003) Understanding chronic pain and the mind–body connection. *Holistic Nursing Practice 17*, 6, 281-287. https://doi.org/10.1097/00004650-200311000-00002

17 Carson, J.W., Carson, K.M., Porter, L.S., Keefe, F.J., Shaw, H., and Miller, J.M. (2007) Yoga for women with metastatic breast cancer: Results from a pilot study. *Journal of Pain and Symptom Management 33*, 3, 331-341. https://doi.org/10.1016/j.jpainsymman.2006.08.009

Crow, E.M., Jeannot, E., and Trewhela, A. (2015) Effectiveness of Iyengar yoga in treating spinal (back and neck) pain: A systematic review. *International Journal of Yoga 8*, 1, 3-14. https://doi.org/10.4103%2F0973-6131.146046

18 McCaffrey, R., Frock, T.L., and Garguilo, H. (2003) Understanding chronic pain and the mind–body connection. *Holistic Nursing Practice 17*, 6, 281-287. https://doi.org/10.1097/00004650-200311000-00002

19 McCracken, L.M. and Eccleston, C. (2003) Coping or acceptance: What to do about chronic pain? *Pain 105*, 1-2, 197-204. https://doi.org/10.1016/s0304-3959(03)00202-1

20 Penman, S., Cohen, S., Stevens, P., and Jackson, S. (2012) Yoga in Australia: Results of a national survey. *International Journal of Yoga 5*, 2, 92-101. www.ncbi.nlm.nih.gov/pmc/articles/PMC3410203

21 Narendran, S., Nagarathna, R., Narendran, V., Gunasheela, S., and Nagendra, H.R.R. (2005) Efficacy of yoga on pregnancy outcome. *Journal of Alternative and Complementary Medicine 11*, 2, 237-244. https://doi.org/10.1089/acm.2005.11.237

ENDNOTES **205**

22 Fishman, L., Saltonstall, E., and Genis, S. (2009) Understanding and preventing yoga injuries. *International Journal of Yoga Therapy 19*, 1, 47–53. https://doi.org/10.17761/ijyt.19.1.922087896t1h2180

23 Le Corroller, T., Vertinsky, A.T., Hargunani, R., Khashoggi, K., Munk, P.L., and Ouellette, H.A. (2012) Musculoskeletal injuries related to yoga: Imaging observations. *American Journal of Roentgenology 199*, 2. https://doi.org/10.2214/AJR.11.7440

24 Swain, T.A. and McGwin, G. (2016) Yoga-related injuries in the United States from 2001 to 2014. Orthopaedic Journal of Sports Medicine 4, 11. https://doi.org/10.1177%2F2325967116671703

25 Russell, K., Gushue, S., Richmond, S., and McFaull, S. (2016) Epidemiology of yoga-related injuries in Canada from 1991 to 2010: A case series study. *International Journal of Injury Control and Safety Promotion 23*, 3, 284–290. https://doi.org/10.1080/17457300.2015.1032981

26 Bachman, R. (2015) Why everyone is a yoga teacher. *The Wall Street Journal*, September 1. https://www.wsj.com/articles/why-everyone-is-a-yoga-teacher-1441128493

27 McCrary, M. (2018) Inside my injury: A yoga teacher's journey from pain to depression to healing. *Yoga Journal*, May 7. www.yogajournal.com/lifestyle/inside-my-injury-a-yoga-teachers-journey-from-pain-to-depression-to-healing

28 Broad, W.J. (2012) How yoga can wreck your body. *New York Times Magazine*, January 5. www.nytimes.com/2012/01/08/magazine/how-yoga-can-wreck-your-body.html

29 Tilbrook, H.E., Cox, H., Hewitt, C.E., Kang'combe, A.R. *et al.* (2011) Yoga for chronic low back pain: A randomized trial. *Annals of Internal Medicine*. https://doi.org/10.7326/0003-4819-155-9-201111010-00003

30 Broad, W.J. (2012) How yoga can wreck your body. *New York Times Magazine*, January 5. www.nytimes.com/2012/01/08/magazine/how-yoga-can-wreck-your-body.html

31 Holton, M.K. and Barry, A.E. (2014) Do side-effects/injuries from yoga practice result in discontinued use? Results of a national survey. *International Journal of Yoga 7*, 2, 152–154. https://doi.org/10.4103%2F0973-6131.133900

32 Penman, S., Cohen, M., Stevens, P., and Jackson, S. (2012) Yoga in Australia: Results of a national survey. *International Journal of Yoga 5*, 2, 92–101. www.ncbi.nlm.nih.gov/pmc/articles/PMC3410203

33 Misra, A. (2014) Common sports injuries: Incidence and average charges. Office of the Assistant Secretary for Planning and Evaluation, March 16. https://aspe.hhs.gov/reports/common-sports-injuries-incidence-average-charges

34 Pappas, E. and Campo, M. (2017) The yoga paradox: How yoga can cause pain and treat it. *The Conversation*, June 29. https://theconversation.com/the-yoga-paradox-how-yoga-can-cause-pain-and-treat-it-80138

35 Le Corroller, T., Vertinsky, A.T., Hargunani, R., Khashoggi, K., Munk, P.L., and Ouellette, H.A. (2012) Musculoskeletal injuries related to yoga: Imaging observations. *American Journal of Roentgenology 199*, 2. https://doi.org/10.2214/AJR.11.7440

36 Mikkonen, J., Pedersen, P., and McCarthy, P.W. (2007) A survey of musculoskeletal injury among Ashtanga Vinyasa yoga practitioners. *International Journal of Yoga Therapy 18*, 1. http://dx.doi.org/10.17761/ijyt.18.1.l0748p25k2558v77

37 Holton, M.K. and Barry, A.E. (2014) Do side-effects/injuries from yoga practice result in discontinued use? Results of a national survey. *International Journal of Yoga* 7, 2, 152–154. https://doi.org/10.4103%2F0973-6131.133900

Penman, S., Cohen, M., Stevens, P., and Jackson, S. (2012) Yoga in Australia: Results of a national survey. *International Journal of Yoga* 5, 2, 92–101. www.ncbi.nlm.nih.gov/pmc/articles/PMC3410203

Mikkonen, J., Pederson, P., and McCarthy, P.W. (2008) A survey of musculoskeletal injury among Ashtanga Vinyasa Yoga practitioners. *International Journal of Yoga Therapy* 18, 1, 59–64. https://doi.org/10.17761/ijyt.18.1.l0748p25k2558v77

38 Masaoka, Y. and Homma, I. (1997) Anxiety and respiratory patterns: Their relationship during mental stress and physical load. *International Journal of Psychophysiology* 27, 2, 153–159. https://doi.org/10.1016/S0167-8760(97)00052-4

39 Lemay, V., Hoolahan, J., and Buchanan, A. (2019) Impact of a yoga and meditation intervention on students' stress and anxiety levels. *American Journal of Pharmaceutical Education* 83, 5, 7001. https://doi.org/10.5688%2Fajpe7001

40 Van der Kolk, B.A., Stone, L., West, J., Rhoes, A. *et al.* (2014) Yoga as an adjunctive treatment for posttraumatic stress disorder: A randomized controlled trial. *Journal of Clinical Psychiatry* 75, 6, e559–e565. https://doi.org/10.4088/jcp.13m08561

41 Thayer, J.F. and Lane, R.D. (2009) Claude Bernard and the heart–brain connection: Further elaboration of a model of neurovisceral integration. *Neuroscience and Biobehavioral Reviews* 33, 2, 81–88. https://doi.org/10.1016/j.neubiorev.2008.08.004

42 Ramírez, E., Ortega, A.R., and Reyes Del Paso, G.A. (2015) Anxiety, attention, and decision making: The moderating role of heart rate variability. *International Journal of Psychophysiology* 98, 3, 490–496. https://doi.org/10.1016/j.ijpsycho.2015.10.007

43 Van der Kolk, B. (2014) *The Body Keeps the Score: Brain, Mind, and Body in the Healing of Trauma.* New York: Penguin.

44 Chang, K.-M., Wu Chueh, M.-T., and Lai, Y.-J. (2020) Meditation practice improves short-term changes in heart rate variability. *International Journal of Environmental Research and Public Health* 17, 6, 2128. https://doi.org/10.3390%2Fijerph17062128

45 Essential Somatics (2021) Thomas Hanna, Ph.D. https://essentialsomatics.com/thomas-hanna

46 Levine, P.A. (1997) *Waking the Tiger: Healing Trauma. The Innate Capacity to Transform Overwhelming Experiences.* Berkeley, CA: North Atlantic Books.

47 Levine, P.A. (2010) *In an Unspoken Voice: How the Body Releases Trauma and Restores Goodness.* Berkeley, CA: North Atlantic Books.

48 Lee, J. (2013) Glen Mills on Usain Bolt and good sprinting technique. *Speed Endurance*, March 20. https://speedendurance.com/2010/01/27/glen-mills-on-usain-bolt-and-good-sprinting-technique

Longman, J. (2017) Something strange in Usain Bolt's Stride. *The New York Times*, July 20. https://www.nytimes.com/2017/07/20/sports/olympics/usain-bolt-stride-speed.html

49 Wikipedia (2023) Motor unit. https://en.wikipedia.org/wiki/Motor_unit

ENDNOTES **207**

50 Purves, D., Augustine, G.J., Fitzpatrick, D., Katz, L.C. *et al.* (eds) (2001) Neuroscience, 2nd edition. Sunderland, MA: Sinauer Associates.

51 Stergiou, N. and Decker, L.M. (2011) Human movement variability, nonlinear dynamics, and pathology: Is there a connection? *Human Movement Science 30*, 5, 869–888. https://doi.org/10.1016/j.humov.2011.06.002

52 Bernstein, N.A. (1967) *The Coordination and Regulation of Movements.* Oxford: Pergamon Press.

53 Hepple, R.T. (2002) The role of O2 supply in muscle fatigue. *Canadian Journal of Applied Physiology 27*, 1, 56–69. https://doi.org/10.1139/h02-004

Chapter 2

1 Story told to me during a meditation retreat with Joseph Goldstein.

2 Lieber, R.L. and Fridén, J. (1999) Mechanisms of muscle injury after eccentric contraction. *Journal of Science and Medicine in Sport 2*, 3, 253–265. https://doi.org/10.1016/S1440-2440(99)80177-7

3 Hortobágyi, T. and Katch, F.I. (1990) Eccentric and concentric torque–velocity relationships during arm flexion and extension: Influence of strength level. *European Journal of Applied Physiology and Occupational Physiology 60*, 5, 395–401. https://doi.org/10.1007/bf00713506

   Abbott, B.C., Bigland, B., and Ritchie, J.M. (1952) The physiological cost of negative work. *Journal of Physiology 117*, 3, 380–390. https://doi.org/10.1113%2Fjphysiol.1952.sp004755

4 Hody, S., Croisier, J.-L., Bury, T., Rogister, B., and Leprince, P. (2019) Eccentric muscle contractions: Risks and benefits. *Frontiers in Physiology 10*. https://doi.org/10.3389/fphys.2019.00536

5 Julian, V., Thivel, D., Costes, F., Touron, J. *et al.* (2018) Eccentric training improves body composition by inducing mechanical and metabolic adaptations: A promising approach for overweight and obese individuals. *Frontiers in Physiology 9*. https://doi.org/10.3389%2Ffphys.2018.01013

6 Crameri, R.M., Langberg, H., Magnusson, P., Jensen, C.H. *et al.* (2004) Changes in satellite cells in human skeletal muscle after a single bout of high intensity exercise. *Journal of Physiology 558*, 1, 333–340. https://doi.org/10.1113%2Fjphysiol.2004.061846

7 Crosier, J.-L., Foidart-Dessalle, M., Tinant, F., Crielaard, J.-M., and Forthomme, B. (2007) An isokinetic eccentric programme for the management of chronic lateral epicondylar tendinopathy. *British Journal of Sports Medicine 41*, 4, 269–275. https://doi.org/10.1136%2Fbjsm.2006.033324

8 Allen, T.J., Jones, T., Tsay, A., Morgan, D.L., and Proske, U. (2018) Muscle damage produced by isometric contractions in human elbow flexors. *Journal of Applied Physiology 124*, 2, 388–399. https://doi.org/10.1152/japplphysiol.00535.2017

9 Babault, N., Pousson, M., Ballay, Y., and Van Hoecke, J. (2001) Activation of human quadriceps femoris during isometric, concentric, and eccentric contractions. *Journal of Applied Physiology 91*, 6, 2628–2634. https://doi.org/10.1152/jappl.2001.91.6.2628

10 Pizza, F.X., Koh, T.J., McGregory, S.J., and Brooks, S.V. (1985) Muscle inflammatory cells after passive stretches, isometric contractions, and lengthening contractions. *Journal of Applied Physiology 92*, 5, 1873–1878. https://doi.org/10.1152/japplphysiol.01055.2001

11 Oranchuk, D.J., Storey, A.G., Nelson, A.R., and Cronin, J.B. (2019) Isometric training and long-term adaptations: Effects of muscle length, intensity, and intent: A systematic review. *Scandinavian Journal of Medicine and Science in Sports 29*, 4, 484–503. https://doi.org/10.1111/sms.13375

12 Pearson, S.J., Stadler, S., Menz, H., Morrissey, D. *et al.* (2020) Immediate and short-term effects of short- and long-duration isometric contractions in patellar tendinopathy. *Clinical Journal of Sport Medicine 30*, 4, 335–340. https://journals.lww.com/cjsportsmed/toc/2020/07000

13 Kubo, K., Kanehisa, H., and Fukunaga, T. (2001) Effects of different duration isometric contractions on tendon elasticity in human quadriceps muscles. *Journal of Physiology 536*, 2, 649–655. https://doi.org/10.1111%2Fj.1469-7793.2001.0649c.xd

14 Fernandes, T.L., Pedrinelli, A., and Hernandez, A.J. (2011) Muscle injury—physiopathology, diagnosis, treatment and clinical presentation. *Revista Brasileira de Ortopedia 46*, 3, 247–255. https://doi.org/10.1016/S2255-4971(15)30190-7

15 James, R., Kesturu, G., Balian, G., and Chhabra, A.B. (2008) Tendon: Biology, biomechanics, repair, growth factors, and evolving treatment options. *Journal of Hand Surgery 33*, 1, 102–112. https://doi.org/10.1016/j.jhsa.2007.09.007

16 Wu, F., Nerlich, M., and Docheva, D. (2017) Tendon injuries: Basic science and new repair proposals. *EFFORT Open Reviews 2*, 7, 332–342. https://doi.org/10.1302/2058-5241.2.160075

17 Zafar, M.S., Mahmood, A., and Maffulli, N. (2009) Basic science and clinical aspects of achilles tendinopathy. *Sports Medicine and Arthroscopy Review 17*, 3, 190–197. https://doi.org/10.1097/jsa.0b013e3181b37eb7

18 Mirkin, G. and Hoffman, M. (1978) *The Sports Medicine Book*. New York, NY: Little, Brown.

19 Reinl, G. (2014) *Iced! The Illusionary Treatment Option*, 2nd edition. Published by author.

20 Laumonier, T. and Menetrey, J. (2016) Muscle injuries and strategies for improving their repair. *Journal of Experimental Orthopaedics 3*, 15. https://doi.org/10.1186%2Fs40634-016-0051-7

21 Chen, L., Deng, H., Cui, H., Fang, J. *et al.* (2018) Inflammatory responses and inflammation-associated diseases in organs. *Oncotarget 9*, 6, 7204–7218. https://doi.org/10.18632%2Foncotarget.23208

22 Lieber, R.L. and Fridén, J. (1999) Mechanisms of muscle injury after eccentric contraction. *Journal of Science and Medicine in Sport 2*, 3, 253–265. https://doi.org/10.1016/S1440-2440(99)80177-7

23 Best, T.M., Gharaibeh, B., and Huard, J. (2013) Stem cells, angiogenesis and muscle healing: A potential role in massage therapies? *British Journal of Sports Medicine 47*, 9, 556–560. https://doi.org/10.1136/bjsports-2012-091685

24 Demonbreun, A.R., Biersmith, B.H., and McNaly, E.M. (2015) Membrane fusion in muscle development and repair. *Seminars in Cell and Developmental Biology 45*, 48–56. https://doi.org/10.1016/j.semcdb.2015.10.026

25 Birbrair, A., Zhang, T., Wang, Z.-M., Messi, M.L, Mintz, A., and Delbono, O. (2014) Pericytes: Multitasking cells in the regeneration of injured, diseased, and aged skeletal muscle. *Frontiers in Aging Neuroscience 6*. https://doi.org/10.3389/fnagi.2014.00245

26 Wu, H., Xiong, W.C., and Mei, L. (2010) To build a synapse: Signaling pathways in neuromuscular junction assembly. *Development 137*, 7, 1017–1033. https://doi.org/10.1242/dev.038711

27 Mika, A., Olesky, Ł., Kielnar, R., Wodka-Natkaniec, E. *et al.* (2016) Comparison of two different modes of active recovery on muscles performance after fatiguing exercise in mountain canoeist and football players. *PLoS One 11*, 10, e0164216. https://doi.org/10.1371/journal.pone.0164216

28 Buckwalter, J.A. and Grodinsky, A.J. (1999) Loading of healing bone, fibrous tissue, and muscle: Implications for orthopaedic practice. *Journal of the American Academy of Orthopaedic Surgeons 7*, 5, 291–299. https://doi.org/10.5435/00124635-199909000-00002

29 Mika, A., Olesky, Ł., Kielnar, R., Wodka-Natkaniec, E. *et al.* (2016) Comparison of two different modes of active recovery on muscles performance after fatiguing exercise in mountain canoeist and football players. *PLoS One 11*, 10, e0164216. https://doi.org/10.1371/journal.pone.0164216

30 Scialoia, D. and Swartzendruber, A.J. (2020) The R.I.C.E. protocol is a myth: A review and recommendations. *The Sport Journal 24*. https://thesportjournal.org/article/the-r-i-c-e-protocol-is-a-myth-a-review-and-recommendations

31 Stovitz, S.D. and Johnson, R.J. (2003) NSAIDs and musculoskeletal treatment: What is the clinical evidence? *Physician and Sports Medicine 31*, 1, 35–52. https://doi.org/10.3810/psm.2003.01.160

32 Dupuy, O., Douzi, W., Theurot, D., Bosquet, L., and Dugué, B. (2018) An evidence-based approach for choosing post-exercise recovery techniques to reduce markers of muscle damage, soreness, fatigue, and inflammation: A systematic review with meta-analysis. *Frontiers in Physiology 9*, 403. https://doi.org/10.3389/fphys.2018.00403

33 Best, T.M., Gharaibeh, B., and Huard, J. (2013) Stem cells, angiogenesis and muscle healing: A potential role in massage therapies? *British Journal of Sports Medicine 47*, 9, 556–560. https://doi.org/10.1136/bjsports-2012-091685

34 Lewit, K. and Simons, D.G. (1984) Myofascial pain: Relief by post-isometric relaxation. *Archives of Physical Medicine and Rehabilitation 65*, 8, 452–456. https://pubmed.ncbi.nlm.nih.gov/6466075

35 Lethem, J., Slade, P.D., Troup, J.D., and Bentley, G. (1983) Outline of a fear-avoidance model of exaggerated pain perception—1. *Behaviour Research and Therapy 21*, 4, 401–408. https://doi.org/10.1016/0005-7967(83)90009-8

36 Vlaeyen, J.W.S. and Linton, S.J. (2000) Fear-avoidance and its consequences in chronic musculoskeletal pain: A start of the art. *Pain 85*, 3, 317–332. https://doi.org/10.1016/s0304-3959(99)00242-0

37 Ishak, N.A., Zahari, Z., and Justine, M. (2017) Kinesiophobia, pain, muscle functions, and functional perforrmances among older persons with low back pain. *Pain Research and Treatment 2017*, 3489617. https://doi.org/10.1155/2017/3489617

38 Kim, G., Kim, H., Kim, W.K., and Kim, J. (2018) Effect of stretching-based rehabilitation on pain, flexibility and muscle strength in dancers with hamstring injury: A single-blind, prospective, randomized clinical trial. *Journal of Sports Medicine and Physical Fitness 58*, 9, 1287–1295. https://doi.org/10.23736/S0022-4707.17.07554-5

39 Ben, M. and Harvey, L.A. (2010) Regular stretch does not increase muscle extensibility: A randomized controlled trial. *Scandinavian Journal of Medicine and Science in Sports 20*, 1, 136–144. https://doi.org/10.1111/j.1600-0838.2009.00926.x

Law, R.Y.W., Harvey, L.A., Nicholas, M.K., Tonkin, L., De Sousa, M., and Finniss, D.G. (2009) Stretch exercises increase tolerance to stretch in patients with chronic musculoskeletal pain: A randomized controlled trial. *Physical Therapy 89*, 10, 1016–1026. https://academic.oup.com/ptj/article/89/10/1016/2737554

Halbertsma, J.P. and Göeken, L.N. (1994) Stretching exercises: Effect on passive extensibility and stiffness in short hamstrings of healthy subjects. *Archives of Physical Medicine and Rehabilitation 75*, 9, 976–981. https://doi.org/10.1016/0003-9993(94)90675-0

40 Page, P., Frank, C.C., and Lardner, R. (2010) *Assessment and Treatment of Muscle Imbalance: The Janda Approach*. Champaign, IL: Human Kinetics.

41 Markos, P.D. (1979) Ipsilateral and contralateral effects of proprioceptive neuromuscular facilitation techniques on hip motion and electromyographic activity. *Physical Therapy 59*, 11, 1366–1373. https://doi.org/10.1093/ptj/59.11.1366

42 Bandy, W.D., Irion, J.M., and Briggler, M. (1997) The effect of time and frequency of static stretching on flexibility of the hamstring muscles. *Physical Therapy 77*, 10, 1090–1096. https://doi.org/10.1093/ptj/77.10.1090

43 Ayala, F., and de Baranda Andújar, P.S. (2010) Effect of 3 different active stretch durations on hip flexion range of motion. *Journal of Strength and Conditioning Research 24*, 2, 430–436. https://doi.org/10.1519/jsc.0b013e3181c0674f

44 Reynolds, G. (2013) Reasons not to stretch. *New York Times*, April 3. https://archive.nytimes.com/well.blogs.nytimes.com/2013/04/03/reasons-not-to-stretch

45 Kistler, B.M., Walsh, M.S., Horn, T.S., and Cox, R.H. (2010) The acute effects of static stretching on the sprint performance of collegiate men in the 60- and 100-m dash after a dynamic warm-up. *Journal of Strength and Conditioning Research 24*, 9, 2280–2284. https://doi.org/10.1519/jsc.0b013e3181e58dd7

Robbins, J.W. and Scheuermann, B.W. (2008) Varying amounts of acute static stretching and its effect on vertical jump performance. *Journal of Strength and Conditioning Research 22*, 3, 781–786. https://doi.org/10.1519/jsc.0b013e31816a59a9

Fletcher, I.M. and Anness, R. (2007) The acute effects of combined static and dynamic stretch protocols on fifty-meter sprint performance in track-and-field athletes. *Journal of Strength and Conditioning Research 21*, 3, 784–787. https://doi.org/10.1519/r-19475.1

46 Fletcher, I.M. and Anness, R. (2007) The acute effects of combined static and dynamic stretch protocols on fifty-meter sprint performance in track-and-field athletes. *Journal of Strength and Conditioning Research 21*, 3, 784–787. https://doi.org/10.1519/r-19475.1

ENDNOTES   **211**

47 Reynolds, G. (2008) Stretching: The truth. *New York Times*, October 31. www.nytimes. com/2008/11/02/sports/playmagazine/112pewarm.html

48 Reynolds, G. (2008) Stretching: The truth. *New York Times*, October 31. www.nytimes. com/2008/11/02/sports/playmagazine/112pewarm.html

49 Zmijewski, P., Lipinska, P., Czajkowska, A., Mróz, A., Kapuściński, P., and Mazurek, K. (2020) Acute effects of a static vs. a dynamic stretching warm-up on repeated-sprint performance in female handball players. *Journal of Human Kinetics 72*, 161–172. https:// doi.org/10.2478/hukin-2019-0043

50 Fletcher, l.M. and Anness, R. (2007) The acute effects of combined static and dynamic stretch protocols on fifty-meter sprint performance in track-and-field athletes. *Journal of Strength and Conditioning Research 21*, 3, 784–787. https://doi.org/10.1519/r-19475.1

51 Blazevich, A.J., Gill, N.D., Kvorning, T., Kay, A.D. *et al.* (2018) No effect of muscle stretching within a full, dynamic warm-up on athletic performance. *Medicine and Science in Sports and Exercise 50*, 6, 1258–1266. https://doi.org/10.1249/mss.0000000000001539

52 Woods, K., Bishop, P., and Jones, E. (2007) Warm-up and stretching in the prevention of muscular injury. *Sports Medicine 37*, 12, 1089–1099. https://doi.org/10.2165/00007256-200737120-00006

53 Acosta-Manzano, P., Rodriguez-Ayllon, M., Acosta, F.M., Niederseer, D., and Niebauer, J. (2020) Beyond general resistance training. Hypertrophy versus muscular endurance training as therapeutic interventions in adults with type 2 diabetes mellitus: A systematic review and meta-analysis. *Obesity Reviews 21*, 6, e13007. https://doi.org/10.1111/obr.13007

54 Breathe factsheet (2016) Your lungs and exercise. *Breathe 12*, 1, 97–100. https://doi. org/10.1183%2F20734735.ELF121

55 De la Motte, S.J., Gribbin, T.C., Lisman, P., Murphy, K., and Deuster, P.A. (2017) Systematic review of the association between physical fitness and musculoskeletal injury risk: Part 2—Muscular endurance and muscular strength. *Journal of Strength and Conditioning Research 31*, 11, 3218–3234. https://doi.org/10.1519/jsc.0000000000002174

56 Monteiro, W.D., Simão, R., Polito, M.D., Santana, C.A. *et al.* (2008) Influence of strength training on adult women's flexibility. *Journal of Strength and Conditioning Research 22*, 3, 672–677. https://doi.org/10.1519/jsc.0b013e31816a5d45

57 Nóbrega, A.C.L., Paula, K.C., and Carvalho, A.C. (2005) Interaction between resistance training and flexibility training in healthy young adults. *Journal of Strength and Conditioning Research 19*, 4, 842–846. https://doi.org/10.1519/r-15934.1

58 Simão, R., Lemos, R., Salles, B., Leite, T. *et al.* (2011) The influence of strength, flexibility, and simultaneous training on flexibility and strength gains. *Journal of Strength and Conditioning Research 25*, 5, 1333–1338. https://doi.org/10.1519/jsc.0b013e3181da85bf

59 De la Motte, S.J., Gribbin, T.C., Lisman, P., Murphy, K., and Deuster, P.A. (2017) Systematic review of the association between physical fitness and musculoskeletal injury risk: Part 2—Muscular endurance and muscular strength. *Journal of Strength and Conditioning Research 31*, 11, 3218–3234. https://doi.org/10.1519/jsc.0000000000002174

60 Ingraham, S.J. (2003) The role of flexibility in injury prevention and athletic performance: Have we stretched the truth? *Minnesota Medicine 86*, 5, 58–61. https://pubmed.ncbi.nlm.nih.gov/15495679

Chapter 3

1 Iyengar, B.K.S. (2005) *Light on Life: The Yoga Journey to Wholeness, Inner Peace, and Ultimate Freedom*. Emmaus, PA: Rodale, p.28.

2 Fisher, J.P., Young, C.N., and Fadel, P.J. (2009) Central sympathetic overactivity: Maladies and mechanisms. *Autonomic Neuroscience 148*, 1–2, 5–15. https://doi.org/10.1016%2Fj.autneu.2009.02.003

3 Romero-Martínez, A., Lila, M., and Moya-Albiol, L. (2022) Sympathetic nervous system predominance in intimate partner violence perpetrators after coping with acute stress. *Journal of Interpersonal Violence 37*, 11–12, 10148–10169. https://doi.org/10.1177/0886260520985494

4 Zaccaro, A., Piarulli, A., Laurino, M., Garbella, E. *et al.* (2018) How breath-control can change your life: A systematic review on psycho-physiological correlates of slow breathing. *Frontiers in Human Neuroscience 12*. https://doi.org/10.3389/fnhum.2018.00353

Edmonds, W.A., Kennedy, T.D., Hughes, P.A., and Calzada, P.J. (2009) A single-participants investigation of the effects of various biofeedback-assisted breathing patterns on heart rate variability: A practitioner's approach. *Biofeedback 37*, 4, 141–146. https://doi.org/10.5298/1081-5937-37.4.141

Lin, I.M., Tai, L.Y., and Fan, S.Y. (2014) Breathing at a rate of 5.5 breaths per minute with equal inhalation-to-exhalation ratio increases heart rate variability. *International Journal of Psychophysiology 91*, 3, 206–211. https://doi.org/10.1016/j.ijpsycho.2013.12.006

5 Yuan, H. and Silberstein, S.D. (2016) Vagus nerve and vagus nerve stimulation, a comprehensive review: Part II. *Headache 56*, 2, 259–266. https://doi.org/10.1111/head.12650

Browning, K.N., Verheijden, S., and Boeckxstaens, G.E. (2017) The vagus nerve in appetite regulation, mood and intestinal inflammation. *Gastroenterology 152*, 4, 730–744. https://doi.org/10.1053%2Fj.gastro.2016.10.046

Johnson, R.L. and Wilson, C.G. (2018) A review of vagus nerve stimulation as a therapeutic intervention. *Journal of Inflammation Research 2018*, 11, 203–213. https://doi.org/10.2147/JIR.S163248

Das, U.N. (2011) Vagal nerve stimulation in prevention and management of coronary heart disease. *World Journal of Cardiology 3*, 4, 105–110. https://doi.org/10.4330%2Fwjc.v3.i4.105

6 Jerath, R., Edry, J.W., Barnes, V.A., and Jerath, V. (2006) Physiology of long pranayamic breathing: Neural respiratory elements may provide a mechanism that explains how slow deep breathing shifts the autonomic nervous system. *Medical Hyphotheses 67*, 3, 566–571. https://doi.org/10.1016/j.mehy.2006.02.042

7 Fumoto, M., Sato-Suzuki, I., Seki, Y., Mohri, Y., and Arita, H. (2004) Appearance of high-frequency alpha band with disappearance of low-frequency alpha band in EEG is produced during voluntary abdominal breathing in eyes-closed condition. *Neuroscience Research 50*, 3, 307–317. https://doi.org/10.1016/j.neures.2004.08.005

Yu, X., Fumoto, M., Nakatani, Y., Sekiyama, T. *et al.* (2011) Activation of the anterior prefrontal cortext and serotonergic system is associated with improvements in mood and EEG changes induced by Zen meditation practice in novices. *International Journal of Psychophysiology 80*, 2, 103-111. https://doi.org/10.1016/j.ijpsycho.2011.02.004

8   Yu, X., Fumoto, M., Nakatani, Y., Sekiyama, T. *et al.* (2011) Activation of the anterior prefrontal cortext and serotonergic system is associated with improvements in mood and EEG changes induced by Zen meditation practice in novices. *International Journal of Psychophysiology 80*, 2, 103-111. https://doi.org/10.1016/j.ijpsycho.2011.02.004

9   Blazer, D.G. and Hybels, C.F. (2010) Shortness of breath as a predictor of depressive symptoms in a community sample of older adults. *International Journal of Geriatric Psychiatry 25*, 10, 1080-1084. https://doi.org/10.1002/gps.2477

10 Kolář, P., Šulc, J., Kynčl, M., Šanda, J. *et al.* (2012) Postural function of the diaphragm in persons with and without chronic low back pain. *Journal of Orthopaedic and Sports Physical Therapy 42*, 4, 352-362. www.jospt.org/doi/10.2519/jospt.2012.3830

11 Reyes del Paso, G.A., Muñoz Ladrón de Guevara, C., and Montoro, C.I. (2015) Breath-holding during exhalation as a simple manipulation to reduce pain perception. *Pain Medicine 16*, 9, 1835-1841. https://doi.org/10.1111/pme.12764

12 Busch, V., Magerl, W., Kern, U., Haas, J., Hajak, G., and Eichhammer, P. (2012) The effect of deep and slow breathing on pain perception, autonomic activity, and mood processing—an experimental study. *Pain Medicine 13*, 2, 215-228. https://doi.org/10.1111/j.1526-4637.2011.01243.x

Jafari, H., Gholamrezaei, A., Franssen, M., Van Oudenhove, L. *et al.* (2020) Can slow deep breathing reduce pain? An experimental study exploring mechanisms. *Journal of Pain 21*, 9-10, 1018-1030. https://doi.org/10.1016/j.jpain.2019.12.010

Chalaye, P., Goffaux, P., Lafrenaye, S., and Marchand, S. (2009) Respiratory effects on experimental heat pain and cardiac activity. *Pain Medicine 10*, 8, 1334-1340. https://doi.org/10.1111/j.1526-4637.2009.00681.x

13 Hamasaki, H. (2020) Effects of diaphragmatic breathing on health: A narrative review. *Medicines 7*, 10, 65. https://doi.org/10.3390%2Fmedicines7100065

14 Hamasaki, H. (2020) Effects of diaphragmatic breathing on health: A narrative review. *Medicines 7*, 10, 65. https://doi.org/10.3390%2Fmedicines7100065

15 Bradley, H. and Esformes, J. (2014) Breathing pattern disorders and functional movement. *International Journal of Sports Physical Therapy 9*, 1, 28-39. https://www.ncbi.nlm.nih.gov/pmc/articles/PMC3924606

16 Hakked, C.S., Balakrishnan, R., and Krishnamurthy, M.N. (2017) Yogic breathing practices improve lung functions of competitive young swimmers. *Journal of Ayurveda and Integrative Medicine 8*, 2, 99-104. https://www.ncbi.nlm.nih.gov/pmc/articles/PMC5496990

17 Okuro, R.T., Morcillo, A.M., Ribeiro, M.A., Sakano, E., Conti, P.B., and Ribeiro, J.D. (2011) Mouth breathing and forward head posture: Effects on respiratory biomechanics and exercise capacity in children. *Journal Brasileiro de Pneumologia 37*, 4, 471-479. https://doi.org/10.1590/s1806-37132011000400009

18 Festa, P., Mansi, N., Varricchio, A.M., Savoia, F. *et al.* (2021) Association between upper airway obstruction and malocclusion in mouth-breathing children. *Acta Otorhinolaryngologica Italica 41*, 5, 436–442. https://doi.org/10.14639%2F0392-100X-N1225

19 Nestor, J. (2020) *Breath: The New Science of a Lost Art.* London: Penguin Books.

20 McDougall, C. (2010) *Born to Run: The Hidden Tribe, the Ultra-Runners, and the Greatest Race the World Has Never Seen.* London: Profile Books.

21 Corrêa, E.C.R. and Bérzin, F. (2008) Mouth breathing syndrome: Cervical muscles recruitment during nasal inspiration before and after respiratory and postural exercises on Swiss ball. *International Journal of Pediatric Otohinolaryngology 72*, 9, 1335–1343. https://doi.org/10.1016/j.ijporl.2008.05.012

Milanesi, J.M., Borin, G., Corrêa, E.C.R., da Silva, A.M.T., Bortoluzzi, D.C., and Souza, J.A. (2011) Impact of the mouth breathing occurred during childhood in the adult age: Biophotogrammetric postural analysis. *International Journal of Pediatric Otohinolaryngology 75*, 8, 999–1004. https://doi.org/10.1016/j.ijporl.2011.04.018

Trevisan, M.E., Boufleur, J., Soares, J.C., Haygert, C.J.P., Ries, L.G.K., and Corrêa, E.C.R. (2015) Diaphragmatic amplitude and accessory inspiratory muscle activity in nasal and mouth-breathing adults: A cross-sectional study. *Journal of Electromyography and Kinesiology 25*, 3, 463–468. https://doi.org/10.1016/j.jelekin.2015.03.006

22 Derrickson, S. (dir.) (2016) *Doctor Strange.* Marvel Studios.

23 Nazish, N. (2019) How to de-stress in 5 minutes or less, according to a Navy SEAL. ForbesLife, May 30. www.forbes.com/sites/nomanazish/2019/05/30/how-to-de-stress-in-5-minutes-or-less-according-to-a-navy-seal/?sh=6e6b52443046

24 Lin, I.M., Tai, L.Y., and Fan, S.Y. (2014) Breathing at a rate of 5.5 breaths per minute with equal inhalation-to-exhalation ratio increases heart rate variability. *International Journal of Psychophysiology 91*, 3, 206–211. https://doi.org/10.1016/j.ijpsycho.2013.12.006

25 Rhinewine, J.P. and Williams, O.J. (2007) Holotropic breathwork: The potential role of a prolonged, voluntary hyperventilation procedure as an adjunct to psychotherapy. *Journal of Alternative and Complementary Medicine 13*, 7, 771–776. https://doi.org/10.1089/acm.2006.6203

26 Miller, T. and Nielsen, L. (2015) Measure of significance of holotropic breathwork in the development of self-awareness. *Journal of Alternative and Complementary Medicine 21*, 12, 796–803. https://doi.org/10.1089%2Facm.2014.0297

27 Rhinewine, J.P. and Williams, O.J. (2007) Holotropic breathwork: The potential role of a prolonged, voluntary hyperventilation procedure as an adjunct to psychotherapy. *Journal of Alternative and Complementary Medicine 13*, 7, 771–776. https://doi.org/10.1089/acm.2006.6203

Chapter 4

1 Zalatimo, O. (2024) Low back pain. *American Association of Neurological Surgeons.* https://www.aans.org/en/Patients/Neurosurgical-Conditions-and-Treatments/Low-Back-Pain

2 IHME (2018) *Findings from the Global Burden of Disease Study 2017.* Seattle, WA: IHME.

ENDNOTES **215**

3   Smith, L. (2023) 39 back pain statistics: How common is back pain? The Good Body, August 30. www.thegoodbody.com/back-pain-statistics

4   Woodham, M., Woodham, A., Skeate, J.G., and Freeman, M. (2014) Long-term lumbar multifidus muscle atrophy changes documented with magnetic resonance imaging: A case series. *Journal of Radiology Case Reports 8*, 5, 27–34. https://doi.org/10.3941%2Fjrcr.v8i5.1401

5   Goodman, E. and Park, P. (2011) *Foundation: Redefine Your Core, Conquer Back Pain, and Move with Confidence*. New York, NY: Rodale.

6   Added, M.A.N., de Freitas, D.G., Kasawara, K.T., Martin, R.L, and Fukuda, T.Y. (2018) Strengthening the gluteus maximus in subjects with sacroiliac dysfunction. *International Journal of Sports Physical Therapy 13*, 1, 114–120. https://www.ncbi.nlm.nih.gov/pmc/articles/PMC5808006

7   Buckthorpe, M., Stride, M., and Della Villa, F. (2019) Assessing and treating gluteus maximus weakness—a clinical commentary. *International Journal of Sports Physical Therapy 14*, 4, 655–669. https://www.ncbi.nlm.nih.gov/pmc/articles/PMC6670060

8   Hadeed, A. and Tapscott, D.C. (2023) Ilotibial band friction syndrome. In StatPearls [Internet]. Treasure Island, FL: StatPearls Publishing.

9   Sadler, S., Cassidy, S., Peterson, B., Spink, B., and Chuter, V. (2019) Gluteus medius muscle function in people with and without low back pain: A systematic review. *BMC Musculoskeletal Disorders 20*, 1, 463. https://doi.org/10.1186/s12891-019-2833-4

Chapter 5

1   OrthoInfo (2020) Total hip replacement. https://orthoinfo.aaos.org/en/treatment/total-hip-replacement

2   Katano, H., Ozeki, N., Kohno, Y., Nakawaga, Y. *et al.* (2021) Trends in arthroplasty in Japan by a complete survey, 2014–2017. *Journal of Orthopaedic Science 26*, 5, 812–822. https://doi.org/10.1016/j.jos.2020.07.022

3   Kim, E.-K. (2016) The effect of gluteus medius strengthening on the knee joint function score and pain in meniscal surgery patients. *Journal of Physical Therapy Science 28*, 10, 2751–2753. https://doi.org/10.1589%2Fjpts.28.2751

4   Distefano, L.J., Blackburn, J.T., Marshall, S.W., and Padua, D.A. (2009) Gluteal muscle activation during common therapeutic exercises. *Journal of Orthopaedic and Sports Physical Therapy 39*, 7, 532–540. https://doi.org/10.2519/jospt.2009.2796

Chapter 6

1   Hartmann, H., Wirth, K., and Klusemann, M. (2013) Analysis of the load on the knee joint and vertebral column with changes in squatting depth and weight load. *Sports Medicine 43*, 10, 993–1008. https://doi.org/10.1007/s40279-013-0073-6

2   Rabin, A., Portnoy, S., and Kozol, Z. (2016) The association of ankle dorsiflexion range of motion with hip and knee kinematics during the lateral step-down test. *Journal of Orthopaedic and Sports Physical Therapy 46*, 11, 1002–1009. https://doi.org/10.2519/jospt.2016.6621

Chapter 7

1   Jahn, S., Seror, J., and Klein, J. (2016) Lubrication of articular cartilage. *Annual Review of Biomedical Engineering 18*, 235–258. https://doi.org/10.1146/annurev-bio-eng-081514-123305

2   Rugg, C.M., Hettrich, C.M., Ortiz, S., Wolf, B.R., MOON Shoulder Instability Group, and Zhang, A.L. (2018) Surgical stabilization for first-time shoulder dislocators: A multicenter analysis. *Journal of Shoulder and Elbow Surgery 27*, 4, 674–685. https://doi.org/10.1016/j.jse.2017.10.041

3   Rosenfeld, S.B., Schroeder, K., and Watkins-Castillo, S.I. (2018) The economic burden of musculoskeletal disease in children and adolescents in the United States. *Journal of Pediatric Othopedics 38*, 4, e230–e236. https://doi.org/10.1097/bpo.0000000000001131

4   Cowan, P.T., Mudreac, A., and Varacallo, M. (2023) Anatomy, back, scapula. In StatPearls [Internet]. Treasure Island, FL: StatPearls Publishing.

Chapter 8

1   Kapreli, E., Vourazanis, E., and Strimpakos, N. (2008) Neck pain causes respiratory dysfunction. *Medical Hypotheses 70*, 5, 1009–1013. https://doi.org/10.1016/j.mehy.2007.07.050

2   Dimitriadis, Z., Kapreli, E., Strimpakos, N., and Oldham, J. (2013) Respiratory weakness in patients with chronic neck pain. *Manual Therapy 18*, 3, 248–253. https://doi.org/10.1016/j.math.2012.10.014

3   Kang, J., Jeong, D.-K., and Choi, H. (2016) The effect of feedback respiratory exercise on muscle activity, craniovertebral angle, and neck disability index of the neck flexors of patients with forward head posture. *Journal of Physical Therapy Science 28*, 9, 2477–2481. https://doi.org/10.1589%2Fjpts.28.2477

4   Kapreli, E., Vourazanis, E., and Strimpakos, N. (2008) Neck pain causes respiratory dysfunction. *Medical Hypotheses 70*, 5, 1009–1013. https://doi.org/10.1016/j.mehy.2007.07.050

5   Ferrari, R. and Russell, A.S. (2003) Regional musculoskeletal conditions: Neck pain. *Best Practice and Research: Clinical Rheumatology 17*, 1, 57–70. https://doi.org/10.1016/S1521-6942(02)00097-9

Chapter 9

1   Added, M.A.N., de Freitas, D.G., Kasawara, K.T., Martin, R.L., and Fukuda, T.Y. (2018) Strengthening the gluteus maximus in subjects with sacroiliac dysfunction. *International Journal of Sports Physical Therapy 13*, 1, 114–120.

2   Added, M.A.N., de Freitas, D.G., Kasawara, K.T., Martin, R.L., and Fukuda, T.Y. (2018) Strengthening the gluteus maximus in subjects with sacroiliac dysfunction. *International Journal of Sports Physical Therapy 13*, 1, 114–120.

3   Richardson, C.A., Snijders, C.J., Hides, J.A., Damen, L., Pas, M.S., and Storm, J. (2002) The relation between the transversus abdominis muscles, sacroiliac joint mechanics, and low back pain. *Spine 27*, 4, 399–405. https://doi.org/10.1097/00007632-200202150-00015

Index

ace bandage bridge pose 193
acetabulum 119, 154
active dynamic stretching 61, 66
active range of motion (AROM) 61
active recovery 54-5
active stretching 60-1
aerobic fitness 67, 68
alignment
    benefits to poses 17
    breath guiding 116
    as component of "bulletproof" body 38-9
    definition 39
    myth regarding perfect 37-8
    poor, as common reason for injury 19
    and variability 42-3
"alignment at all costs" regime 38, 141
alternate nostril breathing 72-3, 91-3
amygdala 76
analgesia 55
anapanasati 34-5
anatomy
    hip 119-20
    knee 139-40
    lower back 101-5
    neck 169-72
    sacroiliac joint and glutes 197-8
    shoulder 153-5
anterior cruciate ligament (ACL) 30, 139
anterior pelvic tilt 104-5, 111, 116
anterior superior iliac spine (ASIS) 107, 113
arms at a T 156-7
asana (physical postures)
    and body's innate intelligence 76
    and breathwork 94-8
    conscious relaxation 40-1
    generating strength in back and spine 39
    increasing parasympathetic activity 74
    Iyengar yoga 28

as limb on yoga path 13
and spirituality 26, 27
teacher trainers overly focused on 20
in United States 14
Ashtanga practice 15, 23, 28, 68
athletes
    breathing and performance 80, 82
    stretching for 59, 66-7
    see also sports conditioning principles
atlanto-occipital (OA) joint 169, 171-2
autonomic nervous system (ANS) 25, 73-4, 76

backbend with blanket/blocks 194
back pain
    diaphragmatic breathing for 78
    due to dengue fever 16
    Iyengar yoga reducing 17
    yoga effectiveness 21
    see also lower back pain
ballistic stretching 61
bhujangasana see cobra pose
Bikram practice 15, 28, 68
bird dog 108-9, 114-15
body
    being in 27-9
    components for creating "bulletproof" 38-9
    learning to breathe into 83-90
    pain causing disconnect 16, 18
    and psychosomatics 29-31
    pushing to great lengths 15
    spiritual bypassing in 35-7
    where to breathe in 83
body composition 67-8
Bolt, Usain 37-8
box breathing 81, 90-3
brachial plexus 153
brain stem 75

217

breath
and diaphragm 72, 77–8, 83
guidelines for working with 82–3
holding 41–2, 78
introduction to 71–2
learning to breathe into body 83–90
as medium for uniting body
and mind 40–1
mindfulness of *see anapanasati*
and nervous system 71, 73–6, 82–3, 93
where to breathe in body 83
breath awareness 39, 40, 43–4, 83
breathing
and athletic performance 80, 82
diaphragmatic and thoracic 78–9
nasal vs. mouth 80–2, 170
breathwork
and asana practice 94–8
cardiac coherent breathing 91
holotropic 93–4
practice of 83–90
teachers 72
when to practice 93
see also pranayama (breath control
and energy management)
bridge pose 46, 47, 193, 199–200
Buddha 26–7, 34, 35, 37, 56–7, 76, 90
Bulgarian split squat 151

camel pose lean backs 146
CAR *see* controlled articular rotation (CAR)
cardiac coherent breathing 91, 93
cardiac muscles 49, 73
central nervous system (CNS) 75
cerebral cortex 75
cervical flexion 171–2
cervical nerves 169–70
cervical rotations supine 190–1
cervical rounding 188
cervical traction from standing
forward fold 189–90
cervical vertebrae 169–70, 172
chair pose 49, 105, 111, 140
chair twist 112
child's pose 95
chin tucks while supine 192
chronic pain 16–19, 29
cobra pose 46, 67, 159
compassion 36–7
compensation 39, 41–2
complementary and alternative
medicine (CAM) 17

concentration 13, 34–5, 83, 90, 91, 120
concentric contractions 50, 51
conscious relaxation 39, 40–1, 43
contract-relax agonist contract
(CRAC) 62, 160, 166
contract relax (CR) 62, 63
controlled articular rotation (CAR) 120,
135–7
coracoclavicular ligament 153
coracohumeral ligament 153
corpse pose 98
with blanket under neck 195
with bolster under knees 138,
147, 152, 160, 167, 202
calves on chair 85, 110, 117
prone 84
seated 89–90
supported 84–8
cow face pose 47, 157
CRAC *see* contract-relax agonist
contract (CRAC)

degeneration 53, 119, 141
delayed onset muscle soreness (DOMS) 56
dengue fever 16
dharana *see* concentration
dhyana *see* meditation
diaphragm 42, 72, 77–8, 83, 170
diaphragmatic breathing 78–9, 80, 83
diaphragmatic function 82
Djokovic, Novak 67
donkey kicks 115, 200
downward-facing dog (down dog)
23, 67, 95, 142–3, 148–9
dynamic stretching 61, 66

eccentric contractions 50, 51
eccentric lunge sit-backs 152
emotional tension, techniques
for releasing 31–2
emotions
and being in the body 27–9
impact 24
and meditation 33
and pain 30–1
and posture 170
and psychosomatic disorders 29–30, 79
relationship to breath 71, 73,
75–6, 78, 79, 91, 94
and spirituality 34, 36–7
variability 43
yoga increasing frequency of positive 18

enlightenment
  as limb on yoga path 13
  myth relating to 15–16
enteric nervous system (ENS) 75

fear avoidance model 58
fear of movement *see* kinesiophobia
    (fear of movement)
FHP *see* forward head posture (FHP)
fibrocartilages 19
fight-or-flight response 25, 29, 74, 76
figure 4 200–1
flexibility
  in Bikram practice 28
  as component of "bulletproof" body 38
  as component of physical aptitude 67, 69
  definition 39, 69
  increasing hamstring 48
  as main reason for practicing yoga 14
  myth relating to 15–16, 57
  stretching for 59, 62, 63
  training 68, 69
  without mobility 40
  yoga as most effective path
      for increasing 69
FMS *see* Functional Movement Screen
    (FMS)
forearm plank 116, 202
forearm plank walks 167
forward head posture (FHP) 170, 172
frequency 48
Functional Movement Screen (FMS) 80

glenohumeral joint 46, 153, 155,
    157, 170, 171, 172, 174
glenohumeral ligaments 153
glenoid fossa 153
gluteal muscles (glutes)
  around hip 119–20
  movement practices 17, 49, 105, 198–202
  strengthening 140, 197–8
  types 102–3
gluteus maximus (GM) 36, 102–4,
    115, 127, 137, 197–8, 200, 201
gluteus medius 56, 102–4, 120,
    127, 137, 138, 199
gluteus minimus 102–4, 120, 127, 137
goddess pose 124
golgi tendon organs (GTOs) 63
gomukhasana see cow face pose
groin release with block 132
gut–brain axis (GBA) 75

hamstrings
  active dynamic exercise 66
  good and bad pain 57
  increasing flexibility 48
  muscles 139, 140
  stretching 59–60, 63–4
  synergistic dominance 102
hands-in-the-air pose 47, 110, 155
happy baby 126–7
heart rate variability (HRV) 25–6, 74, 81, 91
hero's pose 147
hip
  anatomy 119–20
  movement practices 121–38
  muscles surrounding 35–6,
      119–20, 127, 137, 198
  ranges of motion 119
hip CARS 135–7
hip hinge pose 105, 110
hip replacements 15, 16, 33, 38, 119
holotropic breathwork 93–4
homeostasis 40–1, 73–4, 75, 82
HRV *see* heart rate variability (HRV)
humeral head 153
hyperlordosis 104, 115
hypertrophy 68
hypothalamus 76

iliotibial band (ITB) 102–3, 127–8, 137
individuality 45–6
inflammation
  electrical vagal nerve stimulation
      decreasing 75
  and excessive sarcomere strain 50
  overactive SNS linked to increased 74, 79
  as phase of healing 53–4, 55
  post-surgery 40
  of tendon 52
infraspinatus 46, 47, 153–4
injuries
  application of discipline 99
  ballistic stretching increasing 61
  definition 23
  and fear of movement 58–9
  and flexibility 69
  and FMS 80
  inappropriate exercises for 46
  and isometrics 51
  massage of trigger points 56
  meniscal 139
  minor neck 154
  and motor control 40

injuries *cont.*
  and movement 55
  phases of healing 53–4
  and plateauing 48
  popliteus 140
  rotator cuff 154
  some causes of 23, 38, 49, 50
  stretching preventing 59, 67
  tendon 19, 51, 52–3
  and variability 42, 43
  yoga carrying risk of 24
  see also yoga-created injuries
inspiration 99–100
intensity 48
internal rotation (IR) 103, 119, 131, 154
isometric contraction 50–1, 62, 63, 157
Iyengar, B.K.S. 14, 60, 73
Iyengar yoga 15, 17, 20, 28, 37

kinesiophobia (fear of movement) 58–9, 172
knee
  anatomy 139–40
  movement practices 142–52
  myth surrounding 141
Kripalu yoga tradition 17

labrum 19, 31, 153
lateral collateral ligament (LCL) 139
ligaments 139, 153
ligament sprains 53
limbic system 75–6
lion's breath 31–2
locust pose 46
  lower body 107, 113
  upper body 108
lower arm isometric 157
lower back
  anatomy 101–5
  movement practices 105–17
lower back pain
  breathwork for 85–7
  and fear of movement 58
  as leading cause of disability globally 101
  muscles as factors in 102, 103–4
  prevalence 101
  and sacroiliac joint 197
  spending on 101

massage 17, 29, 56, 57, 79
MEAT (movement, exercise,
    analgesia, treatment) 55–6
medial collateral ligament (MCL) 139

meditation
  Buddha's tip on 90
  effectiveness on increasing HRV 26
  as limb on yoga path 13
  overlap with psychotherapy 33
  see also anapanasati
meniscus/menisci 19, 139, 140
mental health 14, 24–6, 30, 75
mindfulness 26–7, 29, 34, 37, 79
mini bridge pose 199–200
motor control
  active stretching 60
  CAR requiring 120
  CRAC requiring 62
  for creating "bulletproof" body 39
  definition 39
  depletion after injury 40
  developing 40–1
  and NeuroKinetic Therapy 41
motor programs 40
motor units 36, 39, 40, 124, 130
mountain pose 96, 97
mouth breathing 80–2, 170
movement and exercise 55
movement practices
  gluteal muscles 198–202
  hip 121–38
  introduction 99–100
  knee 142–52
  lower back 105–17
  neck 173–95
  shoulder 155–67
multifidus/multifidi 39, 102, 104
muscle endurance 80
muscles
  abdominal 101
  in active recovery 54–5
  and alignment 38, 39
  in athletes 66
  back 102–5, 109, 117
  and compensation 41–2
  and golgi tendon organs 63
  hamstring 139, 140
  and inflammation 53–4
  massage of 56
  of neck 169–70, 171, 188
  reciprocal inhibition 60, 101
  in repair/regeneration and
      remodeling phases 54
  of respiration 77–8, 80, 90, 170
  rotator cuff 153–4
  of scapula 154–5
  of shoulder 153, 164, 171

INDEX **221**

and specificity 46–7
and stretching 59–60, 61–2
surrounding hip 35–6, 119–20, 127, 137,
	198
trigger points 56, 103
types of 49–50
understanding 100
and yoga 67–9
see also gluteal muscles (glutes);
	multifidus/multifidi; pectoralis
	minor; quadricep muscles
muscle spindle 62–3
muscle strains 50, 51–2, 62
muscular balance 139, 140
muscular contractions 39, 50–1, 60
muscular endurance 67, 68–9
muscular hypertrophy 48, 68
muscular strength 66, 67, 68
myoblasts 54
myofascial release with ball
	109, 117, 127–8, 137
myofibers 53, 54
myofibrils 49, 54
myosin 49
myotendinous junction 19, 52, 63
myth busting
	flexibility 15–16
	knees should never go past toes 141
	perfect alignment 37–8
	yoga as complete exercise program 67–9
	yoga as panacea for pain 21–2
	yoga healing deepest parts 32–3

90/90 130–1
nadi shodhana see alternate nostril breathing
nasal breathing 80–2, 170
neck
	anatomy 169–72
	movement practices 173–95
neck circles 172, 178–87
neck pain 47, 120, 170–1
neck range of motion assessment 173–7
nervous system
	and breath 71, 73–6, 82–3, 93
	keeping calm 40, 56, 82, 93
	and stretching 63, 66
neural edge 43–4
NeuroKinetic Therapy (NKT) 41–2
niyama (personal spiritual practices) 13, 99
NKT *see* NeuroKinetic Therapy (NKT)
nonsteroidal anti-inflammatory
	drugs (NSAIDS) 55

opioids 16, 17–18, 78
overload 45, 48–9

pain
	acceptance of 18–19
	avoidance of 35
	and compensation 40
	in definition of injury 23
	good vs. bad 56–8
	myth of flexibility reducing 15–16
	myth of yoga as panacea for 21–2
	NKT for treating 41–2
	and psychosomatics 29–31
	sacroiliac joint (SI) 78, 102, 197–8
	and self-compassion 37
	see also back pain; chronic pain;
		lower back pain; neck pain
parasympathetic nervous system
	(PNS) 25, 73–5, 78, 93
passive range of motion (PROM) 61
passive stretching 60
pectoralis minor 77, 153, 154, 155, 171, 176
pectoralis minor stretch on wall
	or floor 158–9, 161–2
perfect alignment *see* alignment
phrenic nerve 78, 170
physical aptitude components 67–9
plank pose 23, 49, 51, 116, 167, 202
popliteus 140
popliteus stretch with chair 144, 149
posterior chain 102
posterior cruciate ligament (PCL) 139
posterior pelvic tuck 104–5, 116, 200, 202
post-facilitation stretching (PFS) 62
post-isometric relaxation (PIR) 56, 62
post-traumatic stress syndrome
	(PTSD) 25, 26, 30, 74, 76
pranayama (breath control and
	energy management)
	history 72–3
	increasing parasympathetic activity 74
	as limb on yoga path 13
	nasal breathing 80, 82
	selection 93
	supported set-up 85
	types of 72, 90–3
	when to practice 93
prasarita padottanasana see wide-
	legged forward fold
pratyahara (sense withdrawal) 13
pre-contraction stretching 62, 63
prefrontal cortex (PFC) 75

private yoga therapy 24
progression 45, 47–8
prone external rotation with
blocks 159–60, 166
prone low back traction 114
prone wall angel 163–4
proprioceptive neuromuscular
facilitation (PNF) 62, 160, 166
psoas 31, 36, 103–4, 120
psoas stretch with chair 106–7
psychosomatic disorders 29, 79
psychosomatic experience 29–31
psychotherapy 33–4, 94

"quad lag" 40
quadratus lumborum (QL) 56, 103–4, 199
quadratus lumborum stretch
on chair 106, 111–12
quadricep muscles 17, 36, 40, 49, 51,
66, 104, 126, 133, 139, 140
quadruped plank 116
quadruped position 108, 115, 136, 200

range of motion
avoiding use of 141
drawback to focusing solely on one 171
FHP decreasing 170
flexibility training 69
grade 1 strains 52
hands-in-the-air pose 155
hip 119
injuries limiting 23
neck assessment 173–7
and neck circles 172
passive and active 61
shoulder and scapula 154
in side-lying abduction 126, 133–4
and stretching 59–60, 61, 63
reciprocal inhibition 60, 63, 101
reclined staff pose 98
reclining hand-to-big-toe pose
as example of passive stretching 60,
61
hip sequence part one 121–2
hip sequence part two 128
increasing hamstring flexibility 48
knee sequence part one 142
working on frontal plane 64, 65
working on transverse plane 64, 65
remodeling 52, 53, 54, 55
repair/regeneration 53–4, 55
repetitive strain injuries 20–1

rhomboid and middle trapezius
lift-offs 162–3
rhomboid stretch 189
RICE (rest, ice, compression, elevation) 53–5
rotator cuff 46, 153–4

sacroiliac joint dysfunction (SIJD) 197–8
sacroiliac joint (SI) 78, 102, 197–8
salabhasana see locust pose
samadhi see enlightenment
sarcomere 49–50
savasana see corpse pose
scapula 153, 154–5, 170–1, 172, 174, 181
"sensory motor amnesia" 29
serratus anterior 154–5
setu bhandasana see bridge pose
short lunge 145
shoulder
anatomy 153–5
movement practices 155–67
side-lying abduction 125–6, 133–4
side-lying external rotation 46
side-lying leg lifts 199
sit to stands on chair 150–1
skeletal muscles 39, 49–50, 54, 55, 74, 77
smooth muscles 49, 73
SNS see sympathetic nervous system (SNS)
somatic experiencing (SE) 29, 94
somatic terminology 29
specificity 45, 46–7
spinal discs 19
spinal traction from hands-
in-the-air pose 110
spiritual bypassing 34–7
in body 35–7
versus compassion 36–7
spirituality
niyama 13, 99
river analogy 82
of yoga 13–14, 26–7, 32–3
spondylolisthesis 21, 46
sports conditioning principles 45–9
see also athletes
sprain/strain 19, 23, 43, 51–2, 53
standing forward fold 96
cervical traction from 189–90
static stretching 60–1, 66
straight arm plank 116, 202
stretching
for athletes 59, 66–7
effect of duration 63–5
and good and bad pain 57

INDEX **223**

nature of 59–60
psoas 103, 106–7
quadratus lumborum 106, 111–12
types of 56, 60–2
of weak muscles 198
and yoga 67
stretch reflex 62–3
supine hip circles with straight
    leg 123–4, 129–30
supta dandasana see reclined staff pose
supta padangusthasana see reclining
    hand-to-big-toe pose
swimmers 164–5
sympathetic nervous system (SNS)
    25–6, 73–4, 75, 76, 79, 93
synergistic dominance 102

tactical breathing *see* box breathing
tadasana see mountain pose
tapas 99–100
teacher training programs (TTPs) 20
tendinosis 52, 64
tendon injuries 19, 51, 52–3
tendons
    adductor longus 132
    of diaphragm 170
    grades of strain 52
    patella 139
    for TFL 137
    see also golgi tendon organs (GTOs)
tensor fascia latae (TFL) 102–3,
    120, 127–8, 137, 199
thoracic breathing 78–9, 80
thoracic extension 171, 172, 177, 187, 194
thoracic flexion 171–2
thoracic rounding 188
thoracic spine 17, 170–2, 174
three-part breath 90, 97, 98
time 48
tissue resilience 42–3
trapezius 56, 77, 154–5, 162–3, 171
treatment 56
trigger points 56, 57, 103
Turkish get up 198–9

upavistha konasana see wide-
    angled seated pose

upper crossed syndrome (UCS) 171, 172
urdvha hastasana see hands-in-the-air pose
ushtrasana see camel pose lean backs
utkatasana see chair pose
uttanasana see standing forward fold

vagus nerve (VN) 74–5, 78
variability 42–3
    body's need for 141
    as component of "bulletproof" body 39
    definition 42
Viniyoga 17
Vipassana
    in Mahasi Sayadaw tradition 18, 33
    in Sayadaw U Ba Khin lineage 35
virabhadrasana II see warrior II pose
virasana see hero's pose

warrior II pose 17, 36, 97, 144–5, 201
weight bearing 23, 48–9, 78, 120, 140, 197
wide-angled seated pose 64, 98
wide-legged forward fold 97

yama (social and ethical guidelines) 13
yoga
    for chronic pain 16–19
    eight limbs of 13
    and flexibility 14, 15–16, 57, 69
    injuries *see* yoga-created injuries
    and mental health 14, 24–6
    myths surrounding 21–2, 32–3, 67–9
    origin of term 13
    as somatic practice 29
    spirituality of 13–14, 26–7, 32–3
    traditional methods of teaching 14
    in the West 13–16, 27
yoga classes
    good and bad pain in 57
    individuality in 45
    vs. private yoga therapy 24
    thoracic extension in 171
yoga-created injuries
    data on 22–3
    myth relating to perfect alignment 37–8
    from physically uneducated approach 15
    rise in 19–21

Acknowledgments

First and foremost, to my mom. Your never-ending love and support has helped me feel safe in this world and fueled my inner journey. I am so grateful for you and love you forever.

To all my teachers: You have helped direct this ship. Without you, I'd still be flailing in the wind.

To my soul friends: JP, Josh, Tim, Démian, Adam, Miah, Nicole, Julie, Josephine, Kaki. Life is so much better with you guys in it. Thanks for being by my side for each and every joy and each and every pain. I love you all.

To Nisachon Xu: You, and your studio in Bangkok are home to me. I am so grateful for our friendship. www.yogasutrathai.com

Tatiana Okuma: Thanks for being such a great model and making the cover of this book shine. May your clothing line (www.gypsyamazon.com) continue to catch fire and spread around the world.

To all my students, past, present, and future: None of this would be possible without you. I am deeply indebted to you all.